Over the Santa Fe Trail to Mexico

Over the Santa Fe Trail to Mexico

The Travel Diaries and Autobiography
of Dr. Rowland Willard

Edited by
Joy L. Poole

University of Oklahoma Press : Norman

*Publication of this book is made possible
through the generosity of Edith Kinney Gaylord.*

✖ ✖

LIBRARY OF CONGRESS CATALOGING-IN-PUBLICATION DATA
Willard, Rowland, 1794–1884.
Over the Santa Fe Trail to Mexico : the travel diaries and autobiography of Dr. Rowland Willard / edited by Joy L. Poole.
pages cm. — (The American trails series ; 25)
Includes bibliographical references and index.
ISBN 978-0-87062-439-1 (hardback)
ISBN 978-0-8061-5751-1 (paper)
1. Santa Fe National Historic Trail—Description and travel. 2. Chihuahua Trail—Description and travel. 3. Willard, Rowland, 1794–1884. 4. Willard, Rowland, 1794–1884—Diaries. 5. Willard, Rowland, 1794–1884—Travel. 6. Americans—Mexico—Biography. 7. Physicians—Mexico—Biography. 8. Medicine—Mexico—Chihuahua (Chihuahua)—History—19th century. 9. Chihuahua (Chihuahua, Mexico)—History—19th century. I. Poole, Joy. II. Title.
F786.W74 2015
917.89′5604—dc23

2015016158

To my mother, Helen Joy Geer,
and author David J. Weber

Contents

Illustrations

Illustrations

Acknowledgments

On one of my first days as a librarian at the New Mexico State Library in 2005, we received a letter from Bonhams auction house in San Francisco, California. Dr. Martin Gammon requested information on a pocket diary to be auctioned by Bonhams. The diary was purported to have been written by Dr. Rowland Willard while he traveled the Santa Fe Trail. Richard Akeroyd, then New Mexico state librarian, asked me to respond to the inquiry. He knew of my interests in western trails and, in particular, my reputation as "mother of the Santa Fe Trail Association." Essentially, Dr. Gammon wondered if New Mexico scholars might be able to verify Dr. Willard's travels in the West. I contacted Dr. Marc Simmons, who knew that a physician by the name of Willard had lived briefly in Taos. I provided Dr. Gammon a favorable response. Coincidentally, in the summer of 2005 I was scheduled to travel to San Francisco, where I had the opportunity to examine and read portions of the diary. I immediately realized it provided new information on early routes, travelers, and international trade activity on the Santa Fe Trail and El Camino Real.

Willard's diary was subsequently sold by Bonhams in 2005 and added to the Western Americana Collection at Yale University's Beinecke Rare Book and Manuscript Library. The following year, I booked a flight to Connecticut and spent the first of many vacations deciphering Dr. Willard's clinical penmanship and transcribing the diary into a digital format. While there, Dr. George Miles, curator of Western Americana, informed me of other interesting materials in the Rowland

and Elizabeth Willard Manuscript Collection. On my second research trip to the Beinecke Library, I discovered that Dr. Willard had written not only a diary but also an autobiography, many decades later. The autobiography expanded on scant information in the diary, which he had written quickly by campfire or in the midst of early morning or noonday sojourns on the trail. Subsequently, on my third research trip, I learned that the Beinecke Library had secured what I called Dr. Willard's return home diary. He recorded his travels across northern Mexico to Matamoros, where in April 1828 he booked passage on a schooner to New Orleans. There, he purchased a ticket on a steamboat to take him home to Saint Charles, Missouri, where his wilderness journey had begun three years earlier.

For their assistance in my own journey to bring the writings of Dr. Willard to light, I gratefully acknowledge the following people and institutions from Missouri: the late Bill Popp and Adam Coward, of the Saint Charles Historical Society; the staff of the Missouri Historical Society in Saint Louis; Santa Fe Trail Association member Mike Dickey, site administrator of the Arrow Rock State Historic Site and State Park; Rod Larson of Arrow Rock; and David Sapp, Booneslick Road Association, Columbia.

The staff of the Beinecke Rare Book and Manuscript Library at Yale offered inordinate assistance during my research there, in particular George Miles and Karen Nagel. I'd also like to extend a special note of gratitude to Dr. Howard Lamar, who graciously offered his encouragement, perspective, and guidance.

Dr. Ben Brown of El Paso, Texas, collaborated with me on research and annotations for several passages pertaining to Mexico. I also benefited enormously from the legacy of publications on the borderlands by the late Dr. David J. Weber of Southern Methodist University. Dr. Weber's guidance and insights provided clues to help identify Dr. Willard's acquaintances. In addition, I would like to acknowledge Clint Chambers, MD, a retired surgeon who is also a member of the Santa Fe Trail Association. He shares my interests in both the Santa Fe Trail and frontier medicine and provided knowledgeable explanations of medicine, treatments, and nineteenth-century conditions.

Early in my career, I had the good fortune to meet Samuel P. Arnold and his second wife, Carrie, at the first Santa Fe Trail Symposium in Trinidad, Colorado. Over the decades I was privileged to share many modern-day adventures along the Santa Fe Trail while attending trail rendezvous or symposia. Our conversations always revolved around western frontier history, including the era of the mountain men, the Bent Brothers and Bent's Fort, trail traders and their merchandise, music, and, of course, food! Holly Arnold Kinney, now proprietress of the Fort restaurant in Morrison, Colorado, continues her family's legacy. Like her father, Holly has a keen interest in western history, which is exemplified by her adept administration of the Tesoro Cultural Center.

Steve Schmidt, David Clapsaddle, and Leo Oliva, scholars who are members of the Santa Fe Trail Association, eagerly responded to my research inquiries. The association, based in Larned, Kansas, is composed of people of all ages and walks of life who are bound together by an interest in the fascinating saga of the trail and the preservation of its many physical traces and landmarks that remain today. Readers are encouraged to join the Santa Fe Trail Association at www .santafetrail.org.

The National Historic Publications and Records Commission and the Association for Documentary Editing in Washington, D.C., provided me with a travel stipend to attend the Institute for the Editing of Historical Documents. Additional funds supporting this research came from Ray and Judy Dewey in their recognition of the importance of the Willard project. I am also grateful to Frank Norris and Brooke Safford, both employees of the Intermountain Long Distance Trails Group of the National Park Service; I worked in partnership with them on two Challenge Cost Share grants awarded by the National Park Service to the associations of the Santa Fe Trail and El Camino Real. The members of the End of the Trail Chapter of the Santa Fe Trail Association also provided valuable research assistance.

I greatly appreciated the camaraderie extended to me by Dr. Rick Hendricks and Rob Martinez from the Office of the New Mexico State Historian. Virginia Lopez and Faith Yoman, librarians of the

Southwest Collection, New Mexico State Library, assisted me tremendously, especially in renewals of my long-overdue books. Chris Mueller provided valuable genealogical research on traders and travelers. Other scholars who assisted me in the final stages of the manuscript included Hal Jackson, Robert J. Torrez, and Joseph Sanchez. Melisa Galvan offered assistance in identifying Matamoros merchants. Richard Salazar, retired archivist from the New Mexico State Records Center and Archives, translated nineteenth-century Spanish documents. Craig Timm and James Wilterding, both physicians, speculated on and deciphered Dr. Willard's nineteenth-century diagnoses and treatments.

I would also like to thank the following: Katherine M. Tassini, librarian for the Haddonfield (New Jersey) Historical Society and her staff; Nancy Mathers of North Carolina, a descendant of Dr. Willard; Luis Urias Hermosillo of Chihuahua, Mexico; Dawn Santiago of Las Cruces, New Mexico; and the staff of the University of Oklahoma Press.

I appreciated the unconditional love and support from my mother, Helen Marie Joy Geer, who during the editing of this book endured an ever-changing medical landscape resulting from her diagnosis of multiple myeloma. Complications from this disease ended my mother's life, as well as that of Dr. David J. Weber. Proceeds from this book will be donated to the International Myeloma Foundation for their work toward discovering a cure.

This book was constructed in phases over a span of nearly ten years. Any false assumptions, omissions, or errors rest with me in my eagerness to introduce this significant early contribution to the scholarship surrounding these western trails. I hope Dr. Willard's travels over the Santa Fe and Chihuahua Trails will spark your interest in learning more about western trails and give you incentive to take your own journey. Happy trails!

Joy L. Poole

Editorial Method

EDITING THESE HISTORICAL DOCUMENTS required numerous decisions in making these nineteenth-century diary passages accessible to modern-day readers. Dr. Willard's penmanship was quite small, a challenge only compounded by his use of pencil and, later, quill and ink. It was sometimes difficult to distinguish between the letters *a* and *o*, *n* and *r*, and a singular letter *u* or an *i*-and-*e* vowel combination. Dr. Willard used capital letters randomly to begin a sentence or a thought, and at other times he may have inserted them for emphasis. When words contained double letters, the acceptable style at that time was to insert a capital letter, for example, *F*, *M*, or *S* in place of *ff*, *mm*, or *ss*. These words have been spelled out with the double letters in the lower case. Dr. Willard also used numerous abbreviations with superscripts, such as "Col" for Colonel or "Spts" for Spirits. Some of these abbreviations have been spelled out, and the superscript letters have been lowered for readability.

Generally Dr. Willard's spelling (or misspelling) of English words did not obscure the intended meaning. However, proper names could be spelled any number of ways, and his Spanish words, especially in the earlier entries, were often spelled phonetically. In many of those doubtful instances, the deciphered word has been placed in brackets or footnoted with an explanatory note to clarify a word or phrase. Some passages that are fully or partially indecipherable have been noted as illegible in square brackets and in some instances partially transcribed.

Punctuation was often lacking in Dr. Willard's diary, so modern punctuation was inserted to assist with legibility. When ending a thought, or more likely for further emphasis, Dr. Willard wrote a dash or underline. To simplify this modern edition, periods are placed at the ends of sentences where it is clear that a complete thought was intended, or to aid the reader's comprehension. Some words also have an underscore in front for additional emphasis, which have been retained. In some cases editorial additions are inserted in brackets to improve clarity of meaning. Because the pocket diary was narrow, Dr. Willard divided many words into syllables at the ends of lines, with an equal sign to indicate continuance on the next line. These equal signs have been removed. Some entries were crossed out by Dr. Willard with a single line. Where possible, these strike-throughs have been deciphered and left intact. Conversely, when he read through his diary years later, he penciled in additional words or names of people, which I have also inserted per his clarification. Some modern punctuation conventions have been applied simply for the sake of consistency, such as placing dollar signs in front of numbers instead of after.

The original format of the diary entries has been modified in favor of a chronicle by the date and/or days of the week. I have aligned the dates and days to the left margin and bolded them for ease of reading. In some passages and instances while traveling, Dr. Willard lost track of the day and/or date. The actual dates or days of the week have been enclosed in square brackets when Dr. Willard did not provide them. In a few cases he wrote two entries on the same day. These double entries have been combined into one.

The autobiography was written sometime after 1867. It was written in ink, with a larger penmanship, on higher-quality paper. The present edition includes only the sections of the autobiography that pertain to Willard's travel experiences on the trails and residencies in Mexico. In the remainder of the autobiography Willard recalls his childhood and his river trip down the Ohio River to the mouth of the Ohio. He provides stories of influential men involved in the formation of Missouri's early territorial government and colorful sketches of life in Saint Charles. After his return to the United States in 1828, he provides information on his travels back east to visit his family. He also describes his business partnerships and career in the Midwest, as well as his marriage and family life.

As with the diaries, the autobiography required a number of editorial decisions in order to ensure readability. Proper nouns have been capitalized, as in negroes to Negroes; arkansas river to Arkansas river; calvary to Calvary. Occasionally, Willard would write a word twice; these duplications have been removed. Dr. Willard's writing generally lacked periods, but he liked to use commas with the word "and" to connect phrases and sentences. It is highly possible that the type of writing implement he used, the absorption quality of the paper, and his physical manner of writing may have resulted in a tendency to leave marks resembling commas rather than periods. When appropriate, periods have been inserted where no punctuation or a comma was used originally. In addition, some uses of "and" or "&" have been eliminated to assist the reader. Finally, the medical terms, medicines, and diseases Dr. Willard describes have been deciphered as faithfully as possible.

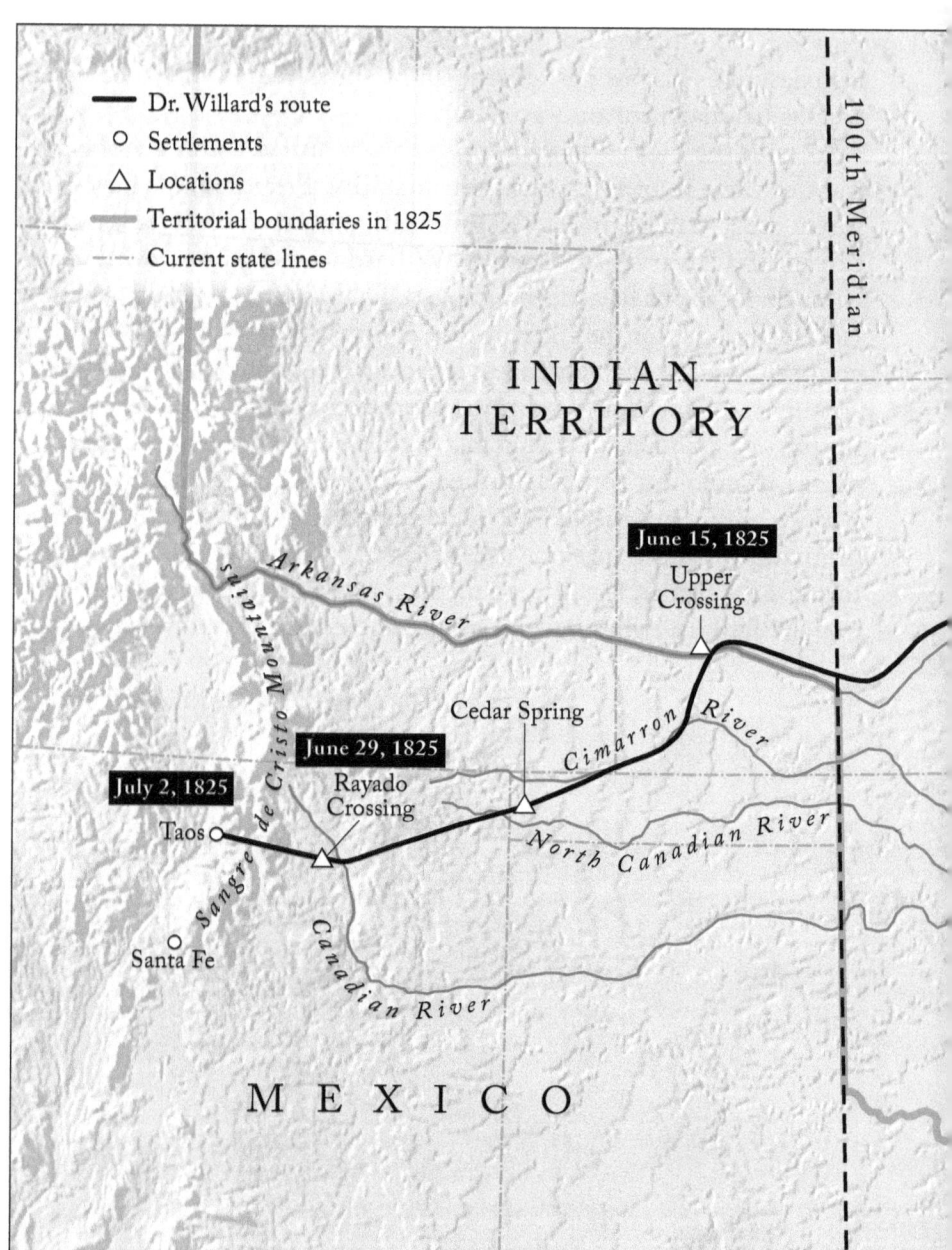

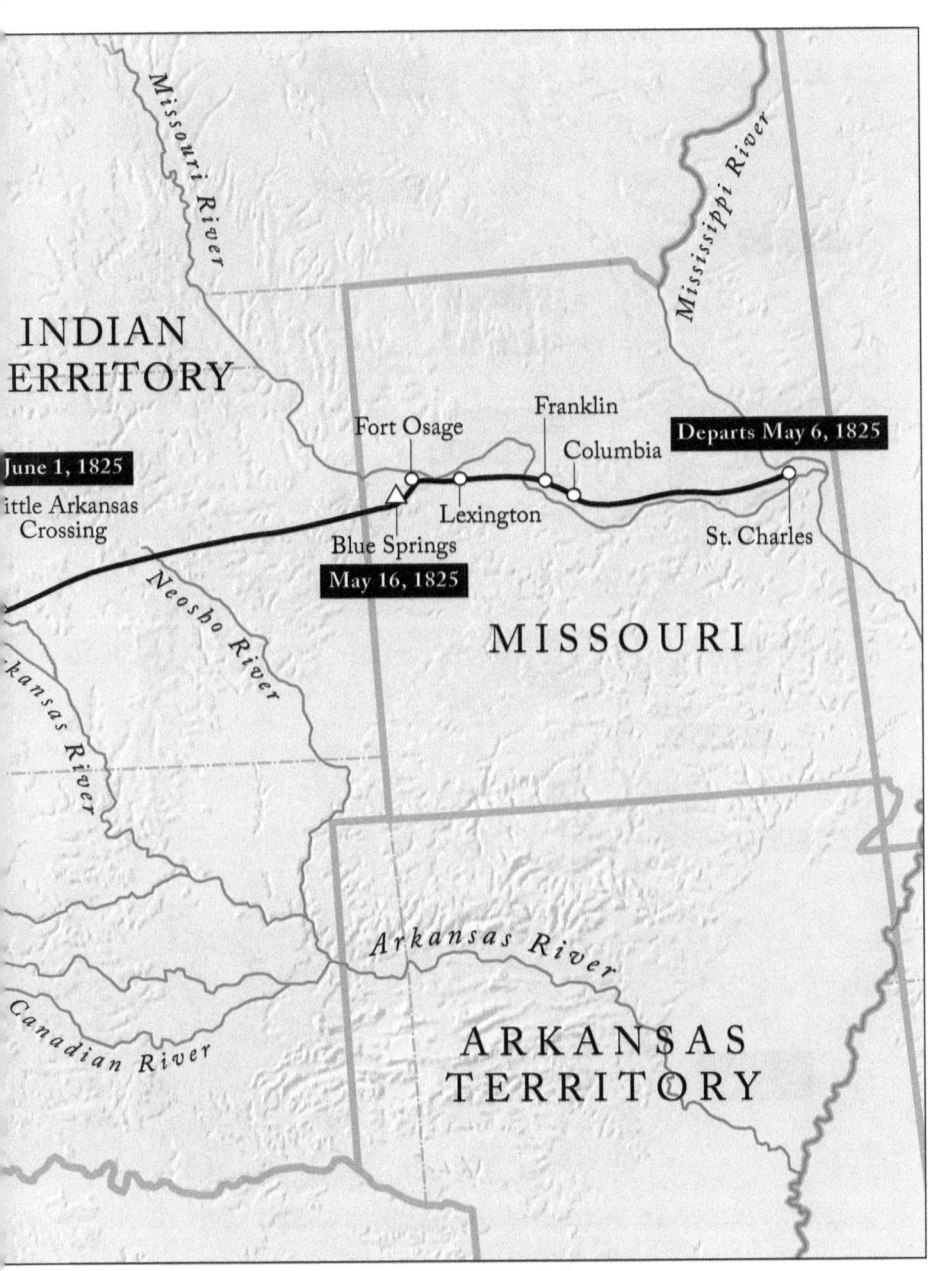

INDIAN
ERRITORY

June 1, 1825

ittle Arkansas
Crossing

Missouri River

Mississippi River

Neosho River

kansas River

Canadian River

Franklin

Fort Osage

Columbia

Departs May 6, 1825

Lexington

Blue Springs

May 16, 1825

St. Charles

MISSOURI

Arkansas River

ARKANSAS
TERRITORY

SANTA FE TRAIL
Willard's route from Missouri through Indian Territory.
Copyright © 2015, University of Oklahoma Press.

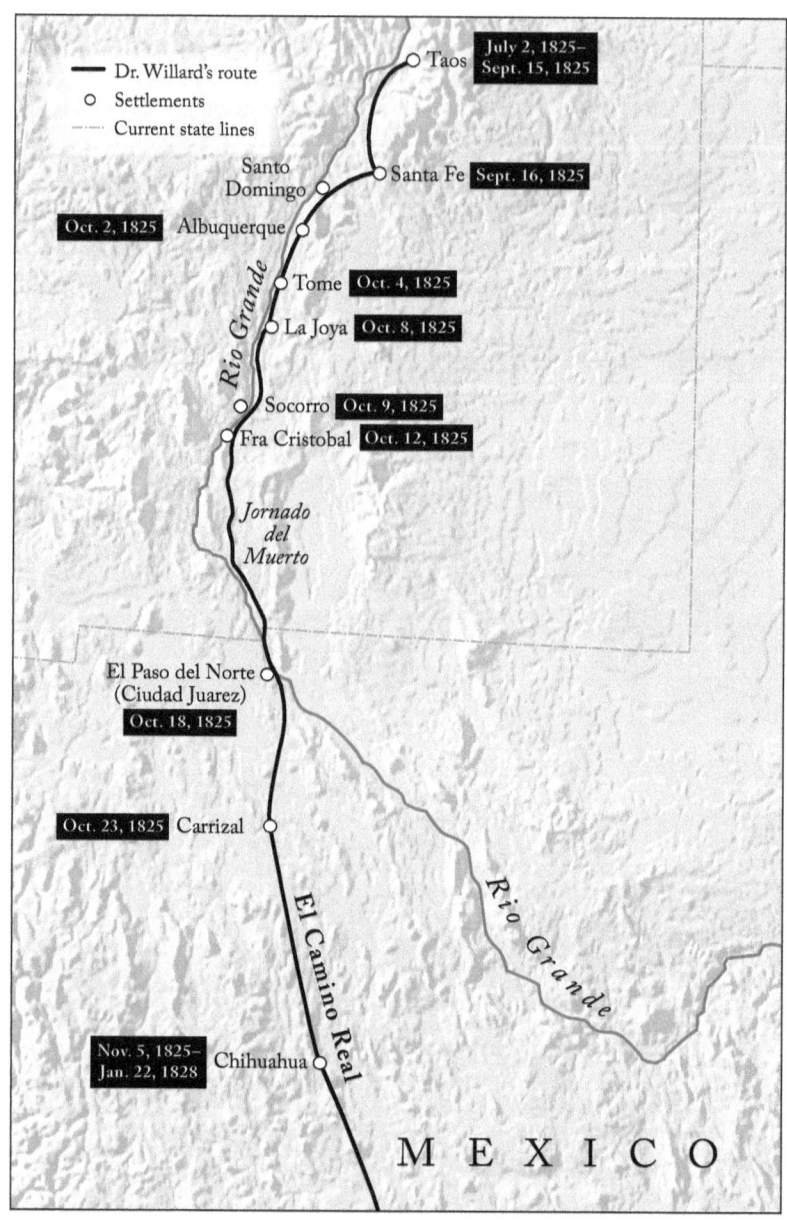

Legend:
— Dr. Willard's route
○ Settlements
-·-·- Current state lines

Taos — July 2, 1825–Sept. 15, 1825

Santo Domingo

Santa Fe — Sept. 16, 1825

Oct. 2, 1825 — Albuquerque

Tome — Oct. 4, 1825

La Joya — Oct. 8, 1825

Rio Grande

Socorro — Oct. 9, 1825

Fra Cristobal — Oct. 12, 1825

Jornado del Muerto

El Paso del Norte (Ciudad Juarez) — Oct. 18, 1825

Oct. 23, 1825 — Carrizal

El Camino Real

Rio Grande

Nov. 5, 1825–Jan. 22, 1828 — Chihuahua

M E X I C O

El Camino Real
Willard's route from Taos to Chihuahua, Mexico,
September 15–November 5, 1825. *Copyright © 2015, University of Oklahoma Press.*

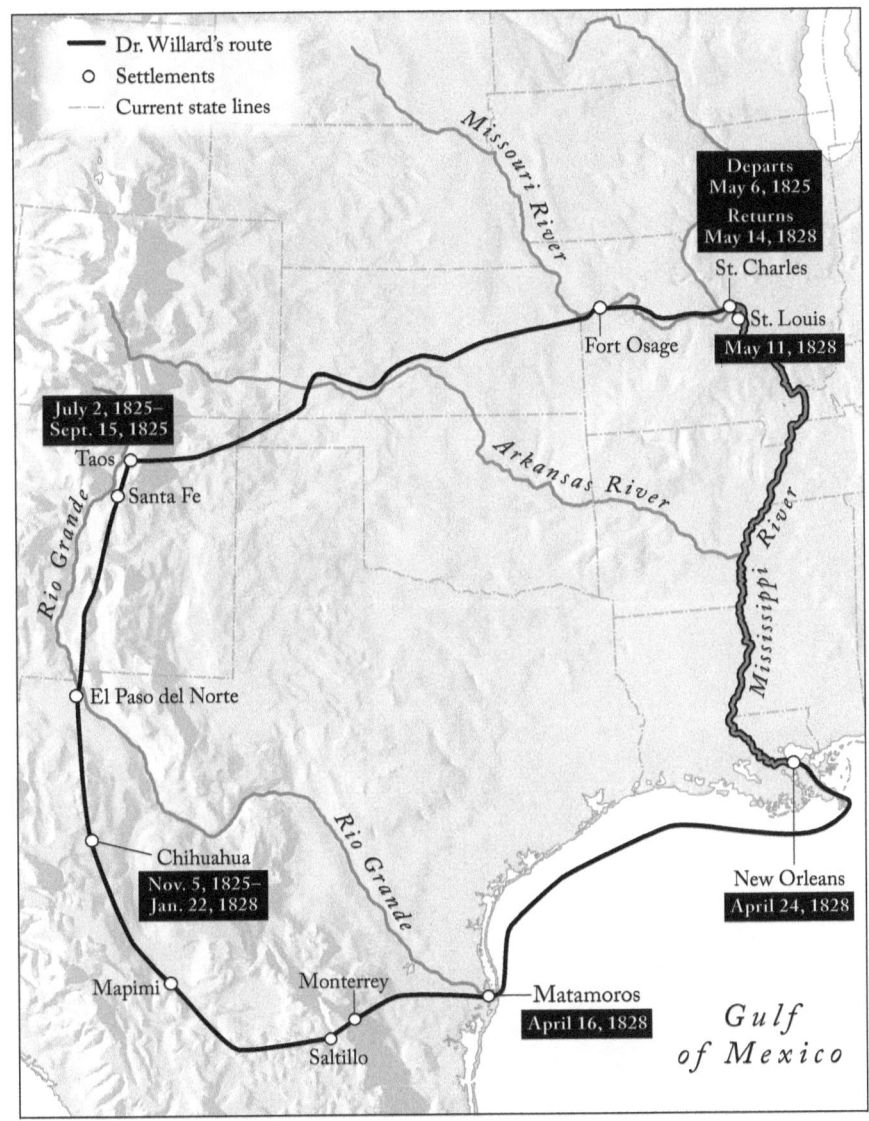

Legend:
- Dr. Willard's route
- ○ Settlements
- — Current state lines

Missouri River

Departs
May 6, 1825
Returns
May 14, 1828

St. Charles

○ St. Louis

○ Fort Osage

May 11, 1828

Arkansas River

July 2, 1825–
Sept. 15, 1825

○ Taos

Rio Grande

○ Santa Fe

Mississippi River

○ El Paso del Norte

○ Chihuahua

Nov. 5, 1825–
Jan. 22, 1828

Rio Grande

New Orleans
April 24, 1828

○ Mapimi

Monterrey ○

○ Matamoros

April 16, 1828

Gulf of Mexico

○ Saltillo

INTERIOR OF WESTERN UNITED STATES
AND NORTHEASTERN MEXICO
Willard's entire route beginning in Saint Charles, Missouri
(May 6, 1825), and ending in Saint Charles, Missouri (May 14, 1828).
Copyright © 2015, University of Oklahoma Press.

Introduction

DR. ROWLAND WILLARD was the first U.S. physician to travel the entire distance of the Santa Fe Trail from Saint Charles, Missouri, to Chihuahua, Mexico. His diaries and autobiography provide a written record of his wilderness journeys over the Santa Fe Trail and down the Chihuahua Trail portion of El Camino Real. His pocket diaries chronicle his daily experiences on a wilderness journey from his home in Saint Charles, Missouri, beginning in May 1825. Sometime after he retired in 1867, Dr. Willard penned a descriptive autobiography that expanded on his diary entries—writings that were hurriedly written while en route or later during brief lulls in his daily practice.

Throughout the spring of 1825, he heard about the formation of an annual Santa Fe Trail expedition to Mexico, and in April he decided to join the foreign adventure. To prepare, Willard purchased two horses, a saddle, and a bridle. Although he had a rifle, he also placed an order for a set of rifle pistols to be made. As he waited for the gunsmith to finish making his pistols, he grew anxious. While he knew the trade expedition had not left the upper settlements of Missouri, there was some urgency if he were to rendezvous with the men gathering at Fort Osage, Missouri, for their departure in May.

Willard had recently completed a medical apprenticeship in Saint Charles. Because he suffered from intermittent fevers caused by malaria, the trip to the Southwest offered a better climate for his health. In addition, he knew of lucrative business opportunities available as a result of commercial trade with Mexico on the Santa Fe Trail, and the ambitious Dr. Willard was eager to make a success of his medical career. In his own words, "I was now tiptoe for adventure."

The 1820s marked the first decade of Missourians' trade on the Santa Fe Trail. At first, many Missouri farmers used pack animals to carry merchandise to Santa Fe. However, by 1824 cargo in larger quantities was transported in wagons. The 1825 caravan Willard joined was divided into two groups. The advance group of men traveling with pack animals was called "packers." The second group traveled slower by wagon. Willard traveled with the packers. They left the Blue River country of western Missouri and followed the Santa Fe Trail until they reached the Arkansas River. There, the packers followed the river for miles until reaching the Upper Crossing where they took the dry Cimarron Route into New Mexico and over the mountains into Taos. In the first decade of the Santa Fe trade many of the packers, after crossing the Cimarron River, followed an old buffalo road from the plains over the Sangre de Cristo Mountains directly into Taos. The road used for centuries by *ciboleros* (Spanish colonial buffalo hunters) or *comancheros* (Mexican traders) was referred to as "the Spanish trace" or "the Spanish trail" by the Americans. The wagons had to continue on the plains around the mountains into Santa Fe.

In Taos the custom house officer waived the import duties on Willard's medicines, and he practiced medicine there for two months. He then traveled south to Chihuahua, where he obtained a business license to open a medical practice. Many of his patients consisted of the aristocracy of Chihuahua, including residents who had been born in Spain. When these *peninsulares* were expelled from Mexico in 1828, Dr. Willard was advised to leave Chihuahua as well. Deciding to return to the United States, he traveled across northern Mexico and departed from the port city of Matamoros before arriving in New Orleans. From there he traveled by steamboat up the Mississippi River to Saint Louis and overland to Saint Charles.

BIOGRAPHY OF WILLARD

Rowland Willard was born in Fort Ann, New York, on August 4, 1794. As a young man he earned a living as a journeyman carpenter. In 1817 nine of his friends—all young men in their twenties—formed an exploring company bound for the western United States, navigating the Allegheny River to the Ohio River. Willard was intrigued and decided to join the group from its starting point in Olean, New York. The men pooled their resources and bought a thirty-foot flatboat to float down the Ohio River. They had no definite plan other than that each man would be at liberty to leave the group and stay at any river community that seemed promising. By the time the group reached the mouth of the Ohio River, the exploring company consisted of three men. Willard and his two companions traded their flatboat for a skiff and successfully navigated upstream to Saint Louis, in Missouri Territory. At that time, the Territory of Missouri was the western frontier of the United States. Willard recorded his seventy-day journey on the Ohio River in a journal, which is unfortunately lost.

Prior to leaving on the Santa Fe Trail, Willard actively participated in the Saint Charles community. He was a member of the local community band, the Masonic Lodge, and the Presbyterian church. He became close personal friends with Missouri's secretary of state, William Pettus, and other politicians and businessmen. Pettus arranged for Governor Alexander McNair to provide Willard a letter of introduction when he left for Mexico. It was designed in the form of a passport bearing the impress of the great seal of the state. According to Dr. Willard, the official document provided incalculable advantage to him afterward in his travels. When Willard returned from Mexico in 1828, he lingered only a day or two in Saint Charles and then headed east to New York to visit his family, whom he had not seen in more than ten years.

While visiting his family he helped them financially by paying four hundred dollars for a deed of land his relatives owned. During the second half of 1828, Dr. Willard attended classes at Jefferson Medical College in Philadelphia. Owing to his strong abolitionist principles, he moved to Cincinnati, Ohio, where he established a medical practice and opened a wholesale drugstore, one of the first west of the Allegheny Mountains. While residing in Cincinnati, he offered his assistance to various Mexican patriots who were living there after being banished from Mexico.

Willard married Elizabeth S. Borland (b. 1814) in Cincinnati on June 27, 1832. After their conversion to the Baptist faith a year later, the couple moved to Covington, Kentucky, where Dr. Willard helped establish the Western Baptist Theological Institute.

Later they moved to Indiana where they purchased a section of land from three Indians and started the town of Oswego, Indiana. Willard practiced medicine and operated a large farm where his house served as a station on the Underground Railroad. He continued to speculate on land, built the Oswego Mills, and served on the board of directors to build the Columbia, Oswego, and Leesburgh Plank Road. When the railroad came through his section of land, he moved to Warsaw, Indiana, where he continued his practice until 1860. The Willards lived in Indiana about nineteen years. Three sons survived childhood: Dr. Lyman W., a physician and surgeon; Dr. Nelson L., a dentist; and Rowland Jr., Ph.D., a pharmacist. Rowland Jr. would eventually own and operate Willard's Pharmacy in Haddonfield, New Jersey, where Dr. and Mrs. Rowland Willard retired in 1867. Willard Sr. died there seventeen years later, at the age of eighty-nine, on March 10, 1884.

The International Trail of Commerce between Missouri and Chihuahua

During the 1820s, a series of events set the lucrative international trade into motion between Mexico and the United States along the Santa Fe and Chihuahua Trails. In August 1821 Missouri was admitted to the United States as the twenty-fourth state. Saint Charles was designated the first and temporary capital of Missouri. Then, in September of that year, Mexico gained its independence from Spain. By November, William Becknell, from Franklin, Missouri, arrived in Santa Fe with pack horses laden with American trade goods, which he marked up and sold at significant profit. The Santa Fe Trail trade was officially open. Fur trappers, farmers, and businessmen in Missouri were eager to earn income from international commerce with Santa Fe. Once the trade caravans were established, the goods brought from the United States disrupted the monopoly Chihuahua merchants had held in supplying New Mexico residents with goods transported along the Chihuahua Trail. Annual expeditions formed from Missouri to Mexico and, to a lesser extent, from Mexico to Missouri. Both the states of Chihuahua, located on the northern frontier of Mexico, and Missouri, then considered the western frontier of the United States, were destined to benefit economically from a symbiotic relationship of burgeoning international commerce.

Though most trade expeditions after 1821 went from Missouri to Mexico, Mexico had an impact on individual Missourians, and their pocketbooks, well into the mid-1800s. America's first financial crisis, the Panic of 1819, had lasted three years. By 1821 the impact of the financial crisis had reached Missouri, resulting in an economic depression. With little money in circulation, Missourians resorted to a bartering system of exchange. The Bank of Missouri, chartered in 1817, suffered financially due to the Panic of 1819 and failed completely in 1822.

While Missouri's economy was faltering, its frontier commerce soon came to rely on silver specie pouring in from Chihuahua as a result of the Santa Fe trade. This currency in the form of Spanish dollars or coins also known as "pieces of eight" was made of precious silver metals from the mines of northern Mexico. The minted coins were recognized by the U.S. government as legal tender through 1857. Once in circulation, the coins saved the economy of Missouri from complete collapse. As trade flourished between Mexico and the United States, beaver pelts, specie, and mules were exported from Mexico to Missouri and beyond.

Meanwhile, Santa Fe and Chihuahua residents eagerly purchased imported cloth from the United States. While wool was available in vast quantities in Mexico, there was no cloth manufacturing available in Santa Fe. Instead, clothing was made of animal skins and coarse homespun wool. Cotton cloth accounted for most of the merchandise transported from Missouri to Santa Fe and Chihuahua in the early days of the Santa Fe trade.[1] Mine owners, bankers, traders, and businesspeople from both frontier regions were able to capitalize on what would become a profitable run on imports and exports between the two nations for the next six decades.

In January 1825 the U.S. government published a report detailing the merchandise traded and transported along the Santa Fe Trail. Most of the information came from Augustus Storrs, a resident of Franklin, Missouri, who had quickly established himself as an authority on the trail. Pablo Obregón, the Mexican minister to the United States, immediately sent a copy of Storrs' report to his government. By March 28, 1825, the Mexican office of foreign relations asked the governors of New Mexico and Chihuahua for their evaluation of Storrs' report. The newly elected governor of New Mexico, Antonio Narbona, refrained from comment, but Governor José de Urquidi of Chihuahua provided the following response to the minister of foreign relations: Trade with the United States would help civilize the New Mexicans, "giving them the ideas of culture which they need to improve the disgraceful condition that characterizes the remote country where they live, detached from other peoples of the Republic."[2] Would-be traders with a keen eye for investing in goods not available to residents in Mexico and willing to take a risk transporting merchandise westward on the Santa Fe Trail could make substantial profits. Storrs' report was an important economic stimulant to ambitious Missouri settlers who needed silver specie and marketable commodities after years of economic depression resulting from the Panic of 1819.

MEDICAL TRAINING AND EDUCATION

Prior to his medical training Willard had worked as a carpenter. The financial depression affected his ability to earn a living, requiring him to evaluate his own financial situation. To gain a steadier stream of income, Willard rented out the brick home he owned on Main

---

[1]Clapsaddle, "Mexican Money/American Commerce," 20.
[2]Weber, *Taos Trappers*, 104.

Street in Saint Charles. After years of struggling with the economic downturn, Willard sold his carpentry tools, having decided, as he phrased it in his autobiography, "to make a transition from physical to mental employment." Dr. Jeremiah Millington had approached young Willard, who had built the doctor's home, with an offer for Willard to study medicine. Jeremiah, along with his brother Seth Millington, had arrived in Saint Charles in 1799. Both Millington brothers were graduates of the University of Pennsylvania's Medical College of Philadelphia, one of the earliest medical schools in the United States. On the frontier, individuals interested in pursuing a career in the medical profession commonly spent three years as apprentices to a medical practitioner. Dr. Millington's generous offer included living quarters on the second floor above Millington's drugstore and post office, which was conveniently located on Saint Charles's Main Street, one block from Missouri's temporary state capitol.

It was not unusual that Millington operated a drugstore as part of his practice. Due to the isolation on the frontier, early doctors were required to be self-sufficient; they often compounded their own medicines from their herb gardens or from plants and roots they gathered. Seth Millington was one of the largest landowners in Saint Charles, where he and Jeremiah had obtained several concessions from the Spanish government. By 1802 they had planted fifty acres of castor bean plants and subsequently opened a castor oil factory employing sixty workers to press beans and bottle castor oil.[3] As Seth continued to farm castor bean plants, he expanded his operations to include mulberry orchards for silkworm production, botanical flower gardens, and medicinal herbs. Beyond their family's drugstore, Jeremiah Millington advertised his services for "Medicine, Surgery and Midwifery" in the newspaper.

From the medical books listed in Willard's autobiography, it appears that Dr. Millington taught according to the instructional method he received at the University of Pennsylvania, using similar medical curricula. Willard studied all the subjects of anatomy, materia medica and botany, chemistry, physiology, pathology, and clinical medicine.

---

[3] The Millingtons sold castor oil to the Lewis and Clark expedition in 1804. Stewart and Knox, *Earthquake America Forgot*, 126.

Willard learned his lessons from medical textbooks while working in Millington's drugstore and serving as the deputy postmaster. The arrangement of working in the drugstore proved beneficial as the pharmaceutical sales improved Willard's business acumen and broke up the monotony of daily studies.

As an apprentice, his anatomy studies were supplemented by two anatomical dissections on human cadavers. During this time, the examination or dissection of corpses was only permitted if they were obtained legitimately. Dr. Millington and his apprentice, Willard, knew both men. The first was Major Mee, who during a time of peace had opened a military school, where Willard enrolled as a student. The major had relied on the military for employment and his income, and the school did not sustain him financially. According to Willard,

> added to these troubles, it appeared in the finale of his career that some family difficulties had annoyed him, & so it was, he retired a few miles in the country where he wrote a short will. Disposing of what he had to several legates & lastly his body to Dr. Millington for dissection, stating that he had endeavored to make himself useful while alive, & desirous to be so after his death, had bequeathed his body for scientific purposes. We sent a man for his remains but they were of little use aside for his bones. He had spoiled his cranium with discharging two pistols through his temples thus immolating himself without cause or purpose.

The cadaver of the other man Willard examined was a French general named Millers who offered Willard fencing instructions. During his first and only lesson, Willard stated,

> while giving me my lesson, he would stand during the pause between the several exercises, & place his forehead upon the hilt of his sword & in broken English say "my head ache very bad." But after taking one lesson of him he took [to] his bed & in some two weeks, died of abscess on the brain. After his death we sawed off the top of his cranium, where we found a cist laying upon the dura mater, containing rather more than a gill of blood. This blood must have been collecting for a considerable time & forming its own receptacle.

Willard, like other American physicians of the time, was influenced by the medical teachings of Dr. Benjamin Rush, who had also taught the Millington brothers at the University of Pennsylvania. Dr. Rush believed that diseases were manifested by fever, "due to the accumulation of a bodily poison that exerted its harmful effect by causing nervous constriction of the small blood vessels. His therapy was designed to rid the body of the poison and to bring about a relaxation of the nervous excitement. . . . Elimination was promoted by bleeding, administering drugs to induce vomiting, purging, sweating, and salivation, and by drawing the poison to the surface by cupping (applying suction cups) and blistering the skin."[4] Rush's widespread and long-lasting influence led Willard to learn the technique of lancing and bleeding his patients and to practice many of Rush's therapeutic methods.

By the time he left Missouri for Santa Fe, Dr. Willard was among a small number of physicians who were well educated, articulate, and learned in the sciences of the day. He was eager to launch a respectable career in a foreign land. At the campsite in Blue Springs, the first day after leaving Fort Osage, he performed a physical examination of the mountain man Hugh Glass, who had been mauled by a grizzly bear nearly two years earlier. Willard's anatomical description of Glass's physical deformities (he called missing sections of Glass's thigh and shoulder blade "chasms") is the only known written and authentic medical record of Glass's injuries. Throughout his travels, Willard routinely treated ailing traveling companions, dispensing drugs from his portable pine medicine chests especially made for the trip.

Once he settled in Taos, the news of the presence of an American doctor quickly spread throughout the little villages of the Taos Valley. His skill as a surgeon was soon established when he performed eye surgery without the benefit of modern-day antibiotics or anesthesia. In his practice, he examined a cross-section of the local population from farm families to the alcalde, or mayor of Taos, to the chief of the Taos Indian pueblo. He frequently notes that patients compensated him with foods they had gathered or grown. Within three months, he realized his goal of a lucrative medical practice was not likely in Taos. The agricultural economy in the northern Mexican frontier, like

---

[4]James E. Bordley, *Two Centuries of American Medicine, 1776–1976* (Philadelphia: W. B. Saunders, 1976), 35.

the Missouri frontier, was based on trade and barter. He discussed his medical career with his American friends as they prepared to return to Missouri with the fall caravan. They advised him to spend the winter in Taos and learn Spanish. The day after they left, Dr. Willard decided to travel farther south into Mexico. He closed his practice and made futile attempts to collect on accounts for his medical services.

With letters of introduction from the governors of both Missouri and New Mexico, he obtained a license and soon established his medical practice in Chihuahua. Coincidently, he had arrived in Chihuahua during a measles epidemic. In fact, one of his patients was his traveling companion, Augustus Storrs, who had recently been appointed as the U.S. consul. In Chihuahua, Dr. Willard soon realized his ambitions to establish a lucrative medical practice. He noted that he examined about twenty patients a day. During his journey and his residencies in Mexico, he only recorded the names of his male patients, their conditions and diagnoses, and the prescribed medicines or treatments rendered. Sadly, he often neglected to record the names of his female patients, referring to them only as the "lady" of Priest _____ or Mr. _____.

Throughout his time in Chihuahua, Dr. Willard experienced an ongoing dilemma. Duties of the Catholic priests included attending to the sick and infirm. Often when a patient's condition was deteriorating, the Catholic family simultaneously summoned Dr. Willard and their priest. Frequently, if the priest arrived first, he had begun to administer the last rites, which included the duties of extreme unction, a healing ritual. This put Dr. Willard in an awkward position for negotiating access to the patient to diagnose and apply his medical ability. It seems, despite both Willard's Protestant-based bias against the Catholic faith and the delicacy of the situation, that he exercised diplomacy.

Overall, his skills as a physician were well regarded, and government officials of Chihuahua asked him to head up a hospital, an assignment he graciously declined. His historical record as the first American physician in northern Mexico identifies a myriad of diseases and illnesses and provides a medical record of the course of treatment prescribed for the time.

THE WESTWARD ROUTE

As the frontier of Missouri was being settled, the Boone's Lick Road led westward from Saint Charles to the beginning of the Santa Fe Trail in Franklin. A map of the Santa Fe route from Missouri was created by Dr. John H. Robinson, who accompanied Zebulon Pike on his 1806 expedition. Residents of Saint Charles owned copies of Pike's 1806 journal, and Robinson's map of Mexico was available to travelers for ten dollars. Willard had likely read Pike's journal, and undoubtedly a copy of Robinson's map was available for those traveling west once they departed from the Boone's Lick Road to rendezvous with those gathering for the annual Santa Fe expedition west. Joseph C. Brown, a surveyor who accompanied George Sibley's exploration of the Santa Fe route in the summer of 1825, also used Robinson's map as a reference. Coincidentally, Sibley had worked with Robinson at Fort Osage and therefore had learned about the route from Dr. Robinson.

Modern-day trail scholars rely on the writing and map from Josiah Gregg's "Commerce of the Prairies," first published in 1844. Gregg, a naturalist, merchant, and author traveled the Santa Fe and Chihuahua Trails multiple times beginning in the 1830s. Dr. Willard's 1825 account of the Santa Fe Trail provides a very early description of the route, campsites, and landmarks of an area not previously explored (or exploited) by annual caravans of traders and merchants. Over time, place names along the route developed from the storied events that occurred at a particular stop, or for their botanical or geological features, a descriptive river crossing, or an available water source. He traveled the route before many of the place names later associated with the Santa Fe Trail were written into the annals of history, and his diaries predate Josiah Gregg's detailed account by nearly twenty years. Willard's writings indicate that his trip was indeed a wilderness journey.

Segments of the Santa Fe Trail parallel the Arkansas River for dozens of miles. Crossing the Arkansas River is frequently described in diaries by trail travelers, who often faithfully recorded their daily miles traveled. One significant point requires further elaboration with regard to the crossing of the Arkansas River. Dr. Willard's firsthand account confirms for trail scholars that the Upper Crossing of the

Arkansas River near present-day Lakin, Kansas, was evidently the preferred and usual route for crossing the Arkansas River throughout the 1820s. Miles of sand hills lined the south side of the Arkansas River. Over time the intermittent flow of Bear Creek cut a drainage channel through the sand hills, leaving a bed of river rock that provided a solid foundation for wagons. Because of Josiah Gregg's 1844 publication, scholars have long assumed that the Middle or Cimarron Crossing of the Arkansas River was the main wagon route. However, the Middle Crossing had a sandy river bottom, which was more hazardous for wagons. Dr. Willard's May 1825 caravan was followed by a wagon caravan captained by Augustus Storrs a couple of weeks later. Both groups crossed the Arkansas River at the Upper Crossing. That same summer, Sibley's exploration party also crossed the Arkansas River at the Upper Crossing.

Willard's autobiography reveals that south of the Upper Crossing, near the Cimarron River, the group of packers encountered an eastbound caravan of Americans and Spaniards. American trader Colonel Meredith Miles Marmaduke and an attorney and businessman from Chihuahua, Don Manuel Simón de Escudero, one of the first Mexican merchants to travel east, were on their way to Missouri.

> Escudero intended to travel no farther than Santa Fe to purchase imported goods from the United States. Happenstance, however, led him to Washington, DC, on an unorthodox international diplomatic venture for the governor of New Mexico. He was sent on a peace keeping mission to address border problems centered on marking a road between Missouri and Santa Fe and defending it against Indians who threatened the security of the traders who used it. For officials in the frontier provinces of New Mexico and Missouri, finding a solution to the problem of Indian raiders was a high priority.[5]

Toward that end, George Sibley's government-sponsored caravan was commissioned to not only survey the road to Santa Fe but also negotiate rights of way for traders with the Osage and Kaw Indian tribes. Sibley's survey party also met Marmaduke's and Escudero's caravan en route to Missouri on July 24, 1825.

---

[5]Weber, "Señor Escudero Goes to Washington," 418.

Another observation regarding the route was that the group of packers, some of whom were mountain men and fur trappers, followed the buffalo trail from the plains directly on to Taos. The buffalo trail was used for both hunting and trading. The packers picked up this "old Spanish trace" from present-day Point of Rocks ranch in northern New Mexico. They headed westward toward present-day Rayado, New Mexico. From Rayado the packers followed the Taos Trail over the foothills crossing the Sangre de Cristo Mountains at Apache Pass,[6] descending into Valle Escondido southeast of Taos and following the Rio Fernandez into Taos.

Publication of Early Travel Journals

Rowland Willard's personal observations are made more revealing through recollections in his autobiography, which he wrote years later sometime before he retired in 1867. It includes his description of the Catholics' reverence for "the Guadalupe," a lively account of a horse race staged by Missouri traders competing with Chihuahua's equestrian owners, and his detailed observations of a traditional bullfight in Mexico. Willard provides new insights into specific Mexican trade items such as the manufacture of coarse hats and the distribution of cigars in Chihuahua.

Upon Willard's arrival in Cincinnati, he loaned his diaries to an acquaintance, Reverend Timothy Flint, a former missionary who had become a well-known regional writer. Timothy Flint's literary reputation resulted from his successful publications about geology and history. These topics were well received by the reading public who were curious about history, the region, and international travel. Willard, who was interested in theology, had first met Flint and heard him preach when he lived in Saint Charles. Subsequently, Reverend Flint, then working as an editor for the *Western Monthly Review*, published excerpts from Dr. Willard's travel diaries in an 1829 essay called "Inland Trade with New Mexico." Willard's travel account was also reprinted in 1831 as an

---

[6]The route Willard traveled confirms the Taos Trail was a spur of the Santa Fe Trail during the first decade of the Santa Fe Trail trade.

appendix to a book Flint edited, *The Personal Narrative of James O. Pattie: The True Wild West of New Mexico and California*. Willard enjoyed a certain amount of fame for his wilderness journey from this publication. In retrospect, it seems appropriate that Dr. Willard's account is included in Pattie's book as he was a contemporary of the Patties and knew both James Pattie and his father, Sylvester. In fact, Willard claimed the Patties visited him in Chihuahua and made their fateful plans for a trapping expedition to California at Willard's home. Ultimately, the trip proved unsuccessful, resulting in the death of the senior Pattie.

Another early travel journal was written by Lieutenant William Hale Hardy of the British Royal Navy. His account of northwestern Mexico, "Travels in the Interior of Mexico 1825, 1826, 1827, 1828," was published in London also in 1829. According to David Weber,

> Hardy entered Mexico shortly after independence had opened the new nation to the relatively free entry of foreigners. Hardy was commissioned by the General Pearl and Coral Fishery Association of England to reconnoiter the potential of exploitation of the Gulf of California and negotiate the appropriate concessions from the Mexican government. At the time, 1825, Mexico was highly interested in overtures made by Great Britain to acquire trade monopolies, and was carefully considering British *versus* United States economic advantages.[7]

Coincidently, Lt. Hardy met Dr. Willard in Chihuahua in 1827 and commented on Willard's social etiquette. It does not appear Dr. Willard knew of Hardy's travel journal, as he does not mention Lt. Hardy or his book in his autobiography written years later.

The only journals Dr. Willard remarks on are those written by Baron Alexander von Humboldt, General Zebulon Montgomery Pike, and Dr. John Robinson, all of whom preceded him into Mexico. Collectively, Willard viewed their works as bearing the character of "literati," especially the publications by Humboldt, given his geological and scientific research.

During the 1820s seven travel journals on Mexico were published in London: six written by Englishmen and one by an American, Joel Roberts Poinsett, U.S. minister to Mexico. All of these accounts, however,

---

[7]Weber, *Extranjeros.*

were derived from and therefore confined to the authors' residencies in Mexico City. Willard's journal of northern Mexico, like Hardy's account, is filled with descriptions of events and characterizations of traders, Mexican and U.S. government officials, Catholic priests, and the genteel society of Chihuahua. A decade later, a number of U.S. travel guidebooks about the Santa Fe Trail trade were published, written by travelers such as Josiah Gregg, Matt Field, Albert Pike, and Alphonso Wetmore. To these widely read and detailed accounts we can now add Dr. Willard's unique American view of the early years of the Santa Fe and Chihuahua Trail trades. Dr. Willard's account describes the early trail trade when it was still speculative, before established routines and standardized merchandise—when the trail trade had not become what Dr. Howard Lamar, professor emeritus at Yale, characterized as "a Conquest of Commerce."[8]

Of utmost importance are the dozens of traders, priests, government officials, businessmen, and residents traced through Willard's encounters with people. Lamar has suggested in his book *The Far Southwest* that the conquest of Mexico was a "conquest by merchants." In his book *The Extranjeros* Weber translated the names of foreign American trappers and traders, based on research at the Mexican Archive of New Mexico that included Santa Fe's customhouse records, the 1826 Report on Foreigners, guías (trade permits), and treasury reports. When taken in combination with these Mexican documents, Willard's authentic personal account naming 170 people is useful in confirming where a trader or trapper was at a specific time.

In summary, Dr. Willard's memoirs provide an authentic account of frontier medicine and the day-to-day activities of residents living in Taos, Santa Fe, and Chihuahua. His revealing characterizations provide insights into the distinctions of class rankings within society, religious and cultural practices, and the various individuals whom he associated with and who benefited from his medical services. Dr. Willard assists the reader in understanding their motivations and personalities, as well as their perceptions and attitudes toward the Santa Fe and Chihuahua trade, Mexico, and its people.

---

[8]Ibid.

Diary 1

May 6, 1825–January 20, 1827

Left St. Charles [Friday] **May 6 1825** at 3 Ock[1] P.M. Rode 9 miles. Put up with Judg Farnsworth.[2] Took a cold cut in the morning and rode to Pond Fort[3] & dined. Put up at Prices[4] having traveled 42 miles.

Sunday [8]. Travelled From Prices to Col. Warners[5] next day, 28 miles.

---

[1] Throughout the diaries Willard uses this abbreviation for "o'clock."

[2] Judge Biel Farnsworth (1772–1847) was one of the original county judges of Saint Charles County, Missouri, when Missouri was established as a state in 1821. Saint Charles County was administered by a panel of three judges. As a county judge, Farnsworth would have been responsible for decisions regarding taxes, road work, law enforcement, and schools. Judge Farnsworth had property nine miles west of Saint Charles in Dardenne Township, on or near the Boone's Lick Road near present-day Cottleville, Missouri.

[3] Pond Fort was one in a series of private forts built as a line of defense during the Indian Wars of 1812. Pond Fort was built by a company of Missouri Rangers under the command of Captain James Callaway. John R. Bell, a member of the Long Expedition, stated that it was "constructed of logs and a square, whose sides are about 200 feet, having block houses at each of the angles, in the interior, and joining to the sides are erected cabins for the accomodation [sic] of families, when they resort to the fort for safety." Bell went on to say that the structure was named Pond Fort because of a large pond two hundred yards north of it. Bell, *Journal of Captain John R. Bell*, 64.

[4] Lemuel Price of North Carolina came to Missouri in 1814 and lived in a fort for a year. In 1815 he and others erected a cabin on the Boone's Lick Road near Camp Branch, in Warren County, Missouri. In June 1825 George Sibley rested for a while at Price's cabin. Sibley notes that the Loutre Prairie beyond Price's cabin was infested with flies, so they waited until sunset before continuing their journey across the prairie. Bryan and Rose, *Pioneer Families of Missouri*, 222; Kate Gregg, *Road to Santa Fe*, 50.

[5] Wynkoop Warner was sheriff of Callaway County from 1820 to 1826. He opened a tavern west of Williamsburg on a variant route of the Boone's Lick Road often referred to in Callaway County court records as the Columbia Road. By December 1825 he was granted a patent *(continued)*

Mare took lame day before consequent to tieing hobbles to tight.
Heavy Shower at 3 reached Warners at dark.

Monday [9]. Leave after breakfast. Several Showers this day. Swapt
My Dory gave $5.00 to boot. Passed Columbia[6] 4 miles. Put up at Mr.
Atkins[7] 28 miles from Warners. Fared hard but well treated. Started
next morning early in the rain. Forded the Persia[8] and breakfasted with
Judge Lyntz.[9] Fared sumptuously. Reached Franklin[10] at sunset after
Swiming 3 creeks and riding in alternate shower all day, dis 28 miles.
Was overtaken by Marble[11] and Knight[12] next morning bound for St.

---

as assignee of Nathan Boone for eighty acres about seven to eight miles west of present-day Williamsburg, Missouri. "General Land Office Records," U.S. Department of the Interior, Bureau
of Land Management, http://www.glorecords.blm.gov/default.aspx (accessed June 7, 2014).

[6]Willard traveled the Boone's Lick Road that was used after 1816 and went from Saint Charles
to Franklin, Missouri. Many of the settlers going west to the Boone's Lick area used this road.
Columbia, the present seat of Boone County, was established as Smithton in 1819 by a group of
settlers. Smithton was moved a bit east in 1822 and renamed Columbia. The original Boone's
Lick Road went north of present-day Columbia. By 1822 travelers headed southwest from Williamsburg along a longer route directly through Columbia, because the growing community
offered amenities. Jackson, *Boone's Lick Road*, 36–37.

[7]Roland Adkins of Boon County obtained a patent on October 1, 1825, for eighty acres. His
property was located where the Columbia Road crossed Perche Creek about four miles west of
Columbia. "General Land Office Records," U.S. Department of the Interior, Bureau of Land
Management, http://www.glorecords.blm.gov/default.aspx (accessed June 7, 2014).

[8]Persia, the creek that Dr. Willard forded, is now Perche Creek. Thwaites, *Early Western Trails*,
147; Williams, *History of Northeast Missouri*, 1:234.

[9]William Lientz (1775–1849) was born in Germantown, Pennsylvania. He and his wife, Mary Miller
Ney Lientz, moved to Missouri from Kentucky. By 1819 they were homesteading four miles
northeast of present-day Rocheport. In August 1821 Lientz served as the foreman of the Boone
Circuit Court grand jury; he was postmaster from 1828 to 1832. Lientz's house served as the post
office until it was moved to Rocheport, in Boone County.*Missouri Intelligencer*, January 1, 1825.

[10]The original starting point of the Santa Fe Trail was Franklin, Missouri. Platted in 1816 on a
low floodplain on the north bank of the Missouri River, the community was named in honor
of Benjamin Franklin. The town was the center of what was called the Boonslick Country,
which stretched over several counties along the Missouri River. In 1821, the year that Missouri
became a state, Franklin became the outfitting point for the Santa Fe Trail. In that year William Becknell departed for New Mexico. A flood in 1828 substantially damaged the principal
commercial district of Franklin. Consequently, businesses and many residents began moving
to higher ground two miles away in what became New Franklin. Simmons and Jackson, *Following the Santa Fe Trail*, 21–22.

[11]On July 8, 1825, Joaquin R. Marble went to the customhouse in Santa Fe and presented a factura
(invoice) dated May 14 from merchandise he obtained in Lexington. Weber, *Extranjeros*, 17.

[12]Robert McKnight (ca. 1789–1846), who was born in Virginia, was an experienced Santa Fe Trail
trader. He joined his brother John and Thomas Brady at Saint Louis in 1809 in a mercantile
adventure. Attracted by Zebulon Pike's published account, McKnight and nine others, including

Fe. Procured several necessaries: 10 lbs crackers 5 lb Beef canteens & ca.[13] Left Franklin at 2 P.M. Traveled 13 miles & put up at Reses[14] 1 mile from the Ferry.[15]

Thursday [12]. Breakfasted at Mr. Smiths. Put up at Davises[16] where we turned our horses out to grass. Rode 30 miles.

Friday [13]. Breakfasted at Mr. Esteses[17] from N. York. Well treated.

James Baird and Samuel Chambers, left for Santa Fe in May 1812. Despite their attempt to open trade with New Mexico, once they arrived in Taos, their $10,000 worth of goods were confiscated and they were arrested as spies. They were taken first to Santa Fe and then to Chihuahua. Their goods were sold. They were assigned to families in Mexico and worked as indentured servants during their confinements in Chihuahua and Durango. A decree freeing the McKnight-Baird party arrived in September 1820. McKnight's brother John went to Durango in 1821 and returned with his brother Robert in 1822. Robert, upon his return to New Mexico, renounced his nationality, became a Mexican citizen, and married in Chihuahua. In May 1825 Robert McKnight traveled west with the packers on the spring caravan from Missouri. McKnight, along with Elisha Stanley, Ira Emmons, and men named Thompson and Shackleford, drew up the company's code of laws for traveling west. In 1828 McKnight gained possession of the Santa Rita copper mine near present day Silver City, New Mexico, where he made a fortune until frequent attacks by Apaches forced him to abandon the mining operation. Josiah Gregg, *Commerce of the Prairies*, 5–7, 12, 56, and Barry, *Beginning of the West*, 119.

[13]"&ca" or "&c" is the equivalent of "et cetera."

[14]George Sibley states in his journal on Tuesday, July 5, 1825; "We crossed the Missouri at the Arrow Rock, and went onto Reece's and Halted. . . . It is 12 miles from Franklin to Reece's." Lewis Rees entered on his quarter section of fertile bottom land near the Missouri River in Miami Township on June 10, 1819, and with others petitioned for the first road in Saline County, leading from Arrow Rock to Grand Pass. Kate Gregg, *Road to Santa Fe*, 52, 249–50.

[15]The Arrow Rock Ferry was located at the narrowest point on the Missouri River, a bit upstream from the present town of Arrow Rock, and was owned in 1825 by Judge David Todd of Franklin (Todd's Landing). In 1820, when the Long Expedition used the ferry, John R. Bell described it as "two canoes, arranged parallel to each other; on these was constructed a platform and railing which was a flooring for our horses and prevented them from going overboard." George Sibley arranged for the team surveying the road to Santa Fe to rendezvous on Tuesday, July 4, 1825, at the Arrow Rock Ferry site. Lawson, "Arrow Rock Ferry," 20–21; Maxine Benson, *From Pittsburgh to the Rocky Mountains*, 74; Bell, *Journal of Captain John R. Bell*, 64.

[16]George Davis from Ross County, Ohio, settled in the Petite Osage Bottom of Saline County in 1816, a little north of the present-day town of Malta Bend. He is said to have planted the first orchard in Grand Pass Township, if not in the county. Missouri Historical Company, *History of Saline County Missouri* (Saint Louis: Missouri Historical Co., 1883), 166–67, 187, 422, 433. Grand Pass, Missouri, is about thirty miles west of Arrow Rock, which coincides with the distance Dr. Willard recorded in his diary. George, along with his son Charles, helped organize the Grand Pass Township of Saline County. Charles married in 1822 and returned by boat to the ferry near present-day Arrow Rock, then overland to Grand Pass Township with his bride, Sallie Kennedy Davis of Chillicothe, Ohio. "Message Boards—Bodkin," ancestry.com (accessed October 20, 2009).

[17]This might have been the same William Estes who resided in Miami Township *(continued)*

Reached Lexington[18] at dusk. Rained most of the day. Rode 30 miles, very muddy. People treated us with considerable attention. Staid next day for Marble & Knight to purchase their goods & lay in such articles as was necessary for this tour: 15 lb. bacon, Tea, Shugar &c.

Left Lexington **Sunday 15th** and overtook the company at Sunset. Some rain this day. Traveled 22 miles. Company in good spirits and consisting of about 90 men & 30 odd waggons. 33 men agree to start next day with pack horses and not wait for the waggons.[19]

Monday 16th. Morning fine. Encamped last night under tent for the 1st time in my life. Took leave of the company[20] and proceeded 10 miles

---

during the first election of Cooper County when it was organized in August 1819. Estes was one of 138 men who voted to elect a delegate to Congress from the territory of Missouri. National Historical Company, *History of Howard and Cooper Counties, Missouri*, 736–37.

[18]Lexington was platted in 1822. The first real significant business was the store and warehouse built by John Aull in 1822. His brothers, Robert and James, followed him in 1825. By 1830 the Aull brothers' stores were selling a wide variety of merchandise to Santa Fe traders. In 1820 they sold between eight and ten thousand dollars' worth of goods to the caravans at 25 percent over Philadelphia prices with no interest for six months and then 10 percent interest until paid. Slusher, "Lexington and the Santa Fe Trail," 6–9.

[19]On this date Dr. Willard arrived at Fort Osage approximately 21 miles from Lexington, Missouri. For a brief period Fort Osage was the westernmost outpost in Missouri. "Fort Osage National Historic Landmark," http://www.fortosagenhs.com (accessed April 19, 2014); Simmons and Jackson, *Following the Santa Fe Trail*, 43–44.

[20]The *Missouri Intelligencer* newspaper published the following account on June 4, 1825, under Santa Fe Adventurers. "We received, the last Western Mail, the following letter, written by one of the Gentlemen composing the company which left this place a few weeks since, on a trading expedition to Santa Fe, in New Mexico.

'Camp near Fort Osage, May 16, 1825
Dear Sir—
We arrived here last evening after a pleasant journey to every respect. Except the rains.—We have been detained several days by different circumstances, mostly by the loss of some horses which we recovered by the badness of the roads, and by the necessity of, building bridges over the mire on each bank of the Big Suiabar [Sniabar]. This being the place of the rendez-vous, the whole company assembled this morning, when the packers concluded, that their strength would justify their going on separately. They have already left us and the wagon company will proceed separately, and under a different organization. The company are in fine spirits, and I have no doubt that their arrangements and conduct will ensure safety. The company here this morning consisted of one hundred and five men, who have thirty four wagons, and above two hundred and forty mules and horses.—Among the packers who are in advance, are Messrs. Morris and Rennison, of Howlud, Mr. Barnes, of Boon, Dr. Willard of St. Charles, and two gentlemen from Natchez. Our code of laws have been prepared by Messrs. Thompson, Stanley Emmons, McNight [McKnight] and Shackelford, a committee for that purpose.—Augustus Storrs was elected Captain, with power, agreeably to the rules, to nominate the subordinate effects and arrange the subdivision of the company.'"

to the blue Springs the place of rendezvous.[21] Some rain. Elected a Captain[22] & Lieutenant[23] R. W. Morris[24] the former & J. Fultcher[25] the latter. Found a plenty of venison at this place killed by some of the company.

---

[21]During the 1820s two routes left Fort Osage. The first forded the Little Blue River six miles west. The second route went south to Blue Spring campground, which was an important rendezvous point. Other traders came to Blue Spring directly from Lexington, and from Cooper, Saline, and Howard Counties. Simmons and Jackson, *Following the Santa Fe Trail*, 45–46.

[22]According to Josiah Gregg, the captain was expected "to direct the order of travel during the day, and to designate the camping-ground at night; with many other functions of a general character, in the exercise of which the company find it convenient to acquiesce." Josiah Gregg, *Commerce of the Prairies*, 31.

[23]The job of the lieutenant was to inspect every ravine and creek on the route, select the best crossings, and superintend what is called, in prairie parlance, the "forming" of each encampment. Ibid.

[24]Robert W. Morris (1800–d. after 1870), an experienced Santa Fe Trail expedition captain, is recorded as one of the American foreigners in the customhouse records of Santa Fe for 1825. Weber, *Extranjeros*, 18. The organization of the expeditions is shown by this announcement, which appeared in an article titled "Santa Fe" in the *Missouri Intelligencer* on March 20, 1824: "Those persons who intend to join the trading expedition to Santa Fe this spring, are requested to meet at Mr. Shaw's tavern, [in Saint Charles, Missouri] on the first day of April next, at 2 o'clock, P.M. to determine whether it will be expedient to pack or convey their goods in small wagons; and to make such other preliminary arrangements as the company may deem proper. A meeting of this kind may be very useful, by creating unanimity with regard to the mode of conveyance and the course to be pursued, and producing uniformity of equipment, which is desirable so far as convenience will permit. I understand that apprehensions of danger from the Indians cause many to hesitate about going. All the information which a strict enquiry has furnished me with, goes to show that no fears need arise from this source. It has been rumored that there is an extensive combination of several Indian tribes against the whites. The naked truth is, that a small band of Osages, being irritated by the frequent intrusion of the people of Arkansas on their best hunting grounds, made an attack on one of these parties who were killing their buffaloe for the hides and tallow, because they could not check this encroachment in any other way. How far they were wrong, is not for me to determine. This however, I believe to be the fact and no circumstances, no other outrages authorize the inference that any tribe whose parties we shall be liable to meet; have a disposition to be at war with the Americans. It is perfectly unreasonable to suppose that they would willingly provoke a conflict, the consequences of which would involve them. In certain and immediate ruin; neither is there evidence that any of them intend it. It will, in my estimation, only be necessary to guard against their stealing, which judicious regulations will almost to a certainty prevent. ROBERT W. MORRIS." Morris was also a licensed tavern keeper and retailer of spirits in Howard County in 1821. Houck, *History of Missouri*, 3:60–61.

[25]Jefferson Fulcher (1787–1859) was born in Amherst County, Virginia. A soldier during the War of 1812, he fought in the Battle of Thames in 1813 where the United States had a decisive victory over British troops and where Shawnee chief Tecumseh was killed. Fulcher moved to Missouri from Madison County, Kentucky, where he married Rachel Stephson on June 16, 1816. By 1821 he was commissioner of Boone County, Missouri. He made several trips to Santa Fe. By 1838 he had moved to Schuyler County, Missouri, where he died in 1859. Goodspeed, *History of Missouri*, 2:1158.

Tuesday 17th. Started at 9 and proceeded 15 miles over ruff country and encamped in a piece of woods when a heavy shower insued with some hail.

Wednesday 18. Travelled 15 mile. Crossed some troublesome creeks and cliffs, bending our course to suit the country.[26]

Thursday 19. Travelled 15 or 18 miles. Was overtaken by 15 or 20 Sack Indians who accompanied us several miles on horseback, appearantly for the purpose of trading horses and skins.

Friday 20th. Travelled 9 miles. Discovered 6 or 8 Elk on the waters of the Caw Riv.[27] Rain insued at 11 ock. where we encamped for the night.

Sunday 22.[28] Rained most of the day yesterday & last night. Cleared away this morning. Two horses broke away last night belonging to Mr. Wallace.[29] They were followed back on the trail 9 miles. Returned without them and Concluded to proceed having pack horses, to carry the goods. The Earth appears completely saturated with water it having rained every day save 2 or 3 since the 6 inst. rained ceased at 9 dried our blankets and started 1/2 past eleven. Saw this day a variety of game consisting of Elk Antelope & Deer. Killed 2 deer only. Travelled 16 or 18 miles and encamped for the night.

Saturday 21st. Prairies appear boundless with occasional thin skirts of timber and should judg this Soil to be second rate tollerably luxuriant producing wild grass and a variety of blossom herbs. All ravines and low grounds contain waters Some of which are crossed with difficulty.

Monday 23d. Started this morning at 1/2 past 7 Ock. Turned out at 10 to wait for a part of our Company which had fel back consequent

---

[26]Dr. Willard is likely on or near the crossing of the Big Blue River in the extreme southwestern corner of Jackson County, Missouri.

[27]Leaving Round Grove, Willard arrived at the Kaw River, now known as the Kansas River, which derives its name from the Kanza or Kaw tribe. It flows through northeastern Kansas. Dr. Willard may have been traveling through Johnson County, Kansas, which lies south of the Kaw River and west of the Kansas/Missouri state line.

[28]Occasionally Dr. Willard's days and dates are out of chronological order.

[29]George Wallit [Wallace] was born in Tennessee in 1793. He became a trader and appeared at the customhouse in Santa Fe. He is listed in the records on July 9, 1825, with a factura issued at Franklin, dated April 25. Weber, *Extranjeros*, 17.

to mules having mired in a creek. When they arrived 2 packs were opened Spread and dried. Started again at 2 making this day 15 miles.

Tuesday 24th. Stood gard[30] last night for the first time warm in the forepart but blew up cold in the latter. The weather seems somewhat more settled this morning than formerly. Traveled this day 20 miles. Saw 2 droves of Elk 20 in each and some Deer. Mr. Glass[31] killed one. No timber this day on the rout but fortunately reached a creek at Sunset where we found a sufficientcy for cooking. This creek is supposed to be a branch of the Virdigree.[32] Prairie exremely wet and troublesome travelling.

Wednesday 25th. Weather appears somewhat precarious though the wind is in a favorable direction. Started at 10. Traveled until 3 ock when we turned out [and] fed the beasts at midday. Saw nothing of importance. Travelled 20 [miles].

Thursday 26th. Started at 9. Crossed 2 bad creeks. Turned out at eleven. Started again at 3 ock. Travelled this day 15 miles. Encamped in Open Prarie without wood. Saw nothing save 1 antelope. Stood guard at night.

Friday 27th. Started quarter past 6 without breakfast. Turned out between 10 & 11. One of the Company killed a fine buck which served

---

[30]Josiah Gregg states, "There is nothing so much dreaded by inexperienced travellers as the ordeal of guard duty. But no matter what the condition or employment of the individual may be, no one has the smallest chance of evading the 'common law of the prairies.' The usual number of watches is eight, each standing a fourth of every alternate night." Josiah Gregg, *Commerce of the Prairies*, 32.

[31]Hugh Glass (ca. 1780–1833) was an American fur trapper and frontiersman noted for his exploits in the American West during the first third of the nineteenth century. "Little is known of Glass until he joined William H. Ashley's fur-trading expedition of 1823 as a trapper. Glass was wounded in the leg during the famous encounter between Ashley's party and the Arikara Indians in 1823. He recovered and joined Major Andrew Henry's party, which set out overland for the Yellowstone River after the fight. While on their way Glass was severely mauled by a grizzly bear at Grand River, South Dakota. He was left behind by two companions John Fitzgerald and James Bridger, who were to guard his final hours. Heartlessly they abandoned him to die, took his rifle, and reported that he was indeed dead. But Glass, according to his own unsupported testimony, crawled many miles down the Grand River, where he joined another party headed up the Missouri. Later Glass journeyed over the Santa Fe Trail where Dr. Willard had the opportunity to examine him." Lamar, *New Encyclopedia of the American West*, 431–32.

[32]Dr. Willard is mistaken. This could be the 110 Mile Creek, which is a tributary of the Kaw River.

us for dinner & supper. Travelled this day 15 miles. One of the hunters reported that he saw 6 or 8 Indians but they did not approach our camp. We lay this night on the waters of the main Virdigress, a tributary to the little Arkansaw.[33] These Streams are skirted with a variety of timbers such as Elm, Lin[den], Sickamore, Coffeenut Honey locust, Swamp oak &c and the adjacent soil exceedingly rich and luxuriant. The prairies produce a variety of herbs such as wild onion, Hog potatoe, wild Tanzy, Siscely, prickly pare &c which are found in great abundance. There are other bub of beautiful flavor and stupour whose names and virtues are to us unknown.

Saturday 28. Some rain last night and this morning partly cleared off at 9. Started at Eleven. Travelled this day 15 miles, 3 out of our way to git to wood and water.[34] Rained insued at Sunset. Saw nothing of importance Save 8 or 10 antelope & Signs of Buffalos.

Sunday 29th. Started at 1/2 past 10 Ock. Traveled 20 miles. Encamped by a litle cotton wood tree the only one in sight. We fel it and with much labour made a fire of its branches. Rain commenced at 11 ock and continued until 7 A.M. and having piched our tent on low ground was discovery made by the rain running under us.

Monday 30. Stood gard the middle wach. Cleared away at 9. Started at 1/2 past 12. Travelled this day 20 miles. Saw signs of Buffalos. Encamped near the Sand Hills.[35] Weather quite cool, grass grows shorter everyday. The prairies here are richly dressed with blossoms of roses and others affording a rich fragrance. Heavy shower passed us this evening.

Tuesday 31st. Morning fine and pleasant. Passed 2 mounds this

---

[33]Given the distance of eighty-eight miles listed in Willard's diary entry of June 1, 1825, and calculated from the main Verdigris to the Little Arkansas, Willard's location is almost certainly the Neosho at Council Grove, Kansas.

[34]The water source would be Diamond Spring, about sixteen miles southwest from present-day Council Grove in Morris County, Kansas.

[35]Willard's distance of thirty-three miles east of the Little Arkansas places him about halfway between Running Turkey Creek and Cottonwood Creek (west of Canton, Kansas; one mile east of the Marion-McPherson county line).

morning constituted of rock resembling Iron ore,[36] Some of which are singularly excavated like Soup dishes, Some hollow with small entrances not unlike Jugs & other vessels. We traveled until 3 ock making about 18 miles and encamped on a small creek where we found a few lovely trees. The prairie is very level and lays fertile than usual. Vegetation appears one month later here than in Missouri.

Wednesday 1st June. Weather fine. A large drove of Buffalos were seen last evening. Mr. Glass is in pursuit of them this morning. Started 1/2 past 7 and traveled to the waters of the little Arkansas,[37] distance 15 miles. The whole face of country we passed today was covered with Buffalos. It would probably be a moderate calculation to estimate their numbers at 100,000 that were seen this fore noon. The hunters brought in a plenty of meat having killed 8 or 10. Dried our Buffalos Soup and stew (without bread) which may be said to be delicious. Passed this fore noon what is called a dog town or a burrough of prairie dogs. They are an animal of the size of a common house cat. Somewhat resembling a dog except their head which resembles that of the squirrel, they sit upon their little univerces formed of the earth they dig from their hole, and when an enemy comes in sight bark vehemently. Their make is rather clumsy, hair short and of a light red colour. They dig their holes so near to each other that they appear domestic and social. Started again at 6 ock follow up the river 3 miles and encamped; after crossing the river Saw 2 Buffaloes which lay mired in attempting to cross it, one of which we endeavored to assist, by putting a rope round his neck and attempting to haul him from his bed but the poor animal was so far spent that he suffered his head to remain under water and drowned. This day has exhibited a great theater of nature. The Buffalos covering the plains as far as vision could extend over a level country, hovering

---

[36]One of the mounds is the site of present-day Jones Cemetery in Marion County, Kansas. The other is a farmstead southwest of Jones Cemetery along the Santa Fe Trail. Steve and Glenda Schmidt own a farm with specimens of iron ore resembling vessels.

[37]Several trail travelers commented on reaching the Little Arkansas, including George Sibley, who wrote in his journal on August 16, 1825, "The Little Arkansas is a clear, brisk running Stream, about 25 yards wide, Water Sweet and good. It is now very Shallow, the bed Sandy, banks high, a few Scattering Cotton Trees along on them. Pretty good pasturage." Kate Gregg, *Road to Santa Fe*, 63.

right and left making way for us to pass. While woolf and antelope were skipping in every direction, exhibited a grand source of reflection and admiration. This park of nature seemed here complete. In front appeared the Sand Hills[38] whose brazen front almost dazzled the eyes, having the appearance of blazing matter from their red complection reflecting the rays of the sun. Travelled 20 miles.

Thursday 2d. Stood gard last night. Shower went round a little before day. Started at 1/2 past 7. Passed several dog towns whose inhabitants are very nervous. Killed 1 Buffaloe. Travelled 20 miles and encamped in open prairie with out wood. Made use of Buffalo dung as a substitute, which answers an excellent purpose. Night cold and windy. Here our bread gave out.

Friday 3d. Started this morning at 8 Ock. Reached the main Arkansas at 10 ck, distance 15 miles. Buffalo as plenty as ever. Killed 4 this forenoon. The Arkansas is a turbid stream from 1/4 to 1/2 mile wide and whose velosity is from 2 to 3 1/2 miles an hour. Its waters I think may be considered wholesome as we could drink almost any quantity without inconvenience. Traveled this day 23 miles. Encamped on the bank of the river.[39] Wind continues high which facilitates our progress as it blunts the scorching rays of the sun.[40]

Saturday 4th. Started at 1/2 past 7. Traveled this morning 10 miles when an unfortunate accident occured. The Buffalo were constantly running before us and sometimes within gun shot. There near approach was to invite the boys sometimes to run out and shute at them. As was the case at this time, myself and several others having curiosity to kill a Buffalo

---

[38]In his 1989 book *Maps of the Santa Fe Trail*, Gregory Franzwa wrote, "Three enormous sand mounds, the Plum Buttes, were two miles to the west. They were well-known trail landmarks. The Kansas winds formed them, and within the last century have blown them away. Only small sand dunes and some plum bushes remain at the site" (80). Matt Field, in his 1843 journal, recorded Spanish names (and translations) for Kansas places; he called the hills Punta la Circuila (Plum Buttes). "Jueves, 17th Left the Arkansas at 6 A.M. Passed a bad mud creek at 7. Punta la Circuila [Plum Point] at 9." Barry, *Beginning of the West*, 383; Field, *Matt Field*, 57.
[39]The Arkansas River.
[40]The site of present-day Ellinwood, Kansas. Santa Fe Trail travelers would have followed the trail and camped along the north bank of the Arkansas River just downstream from Great Bend, Kansas. Franzwa, *Maps*, 86–87.

left our horses and ran forward to get a shot and in so doing turned their course ~~of the Buffalo~~ in the direction of the company and as they passed in front, six pack horses broke from the ranks, fel in with the Buffalo and went off in full speed. They were pursued by 5 or 6 riders who after chasing them 8 or 10 miles caught all but 3 which mixed with the Buffalo and were not afterward seen. These three horses were the property of one man and had on them all his goods (and 300 dollars), provisions and most of his clothing. Myself and another pursued them as soon as we could dispose of our pack horses. We traveled 8 miles in the direction they ran but discovering nothing of them returned. In the evening 7 of us volunteered to go again in pursuit of them. We started a little before sunset. Travelled 8 miles and encamped. Heavy showers ensued at dark. Came upon their track just before dark [and] found they had bent their course up the river. My horse and another broke loose by loosing off the hobbles and made off in the direction of the main camp. Mr. Cave[41] and myself followed them immediately it being 3 Ock at night and tollerable dark. Lost sight of them. We had probibly travelled 3 miles in the direction of this main company when we indistinctly heard the sound of a human voice; and on listening heard it repeated ~~and~~ in the direction of the company we had left. We after a moments consultation, concluded to return to learn the cause. We accordingly made for our camp[42] & on coming in sight (it then being daylight) discovered our horses—who had returned before us.

Sunday 5th. Broiled a peace of meat which constituted our breakfast and again pursued our course. We travelled 7 miles up the river but without success having got hungry and fatigued returned to camp.

[41]Henry Cave (1790–1847), a lawyer, was born in England. Dr. Willard referred to him as L Cave, the L referring to his occupation. He is listed in 1825 as receiving compensation of five dollars from Boon[e] County for his service as a commissioner to view a road in 1822. In the same issue of the newspaper, there is a notice regarding his legal administration of the estate of David C. Westerfield. The notice is signed "Henry B. Cave Jr. Adm's" thus indicating that the widow, Mildred B. Westerfield, hired him as her attorney. *Missouri Intelligencer,* January 1, 1825. As a result of his profitable trip to Santa Fe in 1825, Henry Cave purchased 99.86 acres in Boone County, Missouri, and filed his land claim in the Franklin land office. U.S. General Land Office Records, 1796–1907, ancestry.com (accessed October 29, 2013).

[42]This camp is Walnut Creek Crossing. Matt Field wrote that he crossed Walnut Creek in October 1843. "Miercoles 16th Crossed El Rio de Nuezes [Walnet Creek] without any trouble." Field, *Matt Field,* 56.

Monday 6th. ~~conclude to return to camp~~ pursue our journey. Send out 2 or 3 men nearly on the cours of the river who are to meet us ahead. Rained last night & this morning. Travel this day 22 miles and encamped. All the company arrive but Andrews who we suppose to be loss. Mr. Fulcher to whom the lost horses & goods belong ~~to~~ talks of returning to Missouri. The company endeavor to persuade him to continue and at the same time raised a subscription of $145 to renumerate in some measure his loss.

Tuesday 7th. Marble and Knight fall out, divide their goods, and cause me much trouble. Wind usualy in the south Breezed up from the North. Started this morning at 1/2 past 8. Traveled eight miles when we came to the Pawnee Creek.[43] Obliged to build a raft for the goods and swim the animals. Mr. Fulcher resumes the resolution of returning home. One of the company furnish him with a horse, others with provisions for the tour.[44] Company generaly write by him.[45]

Wednesday 8th. Morning fine. Yesterday winds have mostly subsided. Built fires and shot guns last evening for the guidance of Andrews who has not yet returned. Started at 1/2 past 7. Traveled 20 ms. Encamped on the Arkansas.

Thursday 9th. Started at 1/2 past 6. Wind high. Grass very Short. Buffalo plenty. Travelled 24 miles and encamped on the river.[46]

Friday 10th. Started at 1/2 past 6. Wind high last night and this morning. Traveled this day 25 miles. Encamped on the river.[47]

Saturday 11th. Started at 7. No wind, afternoon quite sultry. Passed 2 volts[48] where a company *cashed*[49] their goods 2 years ago. Consequent

---

[43]Pawnee Creek, Pawnee Fork, and Pawnee River are all the same body of water on the Wet Route near present-day Larned, Kansas.

[44]They apparently camped eight miles west of Coon Creek Crossing, roughly three miles northeast of Kinsley.

[45]The group collectively wrote letters to send home with Mr. Fulcher.

[46]Willard is northeast of the south bend of the Arkansas River.

[47]Dr. Willard would have camped on the eastern edge of present-day Dodge City, Kansas.

[48]Vaults refers to holes in the prairie where goods could be stored.

[49]French Canadian traders and fur trappers originated the term "cache," or a hiding place. "The Caches were made by James Baird and his party of about fifty men, who had set out from

to having lost their mules in a violent snow storm and were obliged to remain through the winter and in the spring go to the settlement for more. Passed the Island where the company last year laid in their meat; traveled this day 24 miles encamped on the river.[50]

Sunday 12th. Heavy dew last night and thick fog this morning. Started at 7, nooned at 10 when a heavy shower commenced with Thunder, lightning and hail, driven with a Strong South wind, which continued to shift its course until it had blown from every direction. Conclude to stay until morning. The Hunters shot 4 Buffalo today. Have thought much of the sweets of domestic life. Though my mind is perfectly tranquil and resigned to endure the privations incident to a long wilderness journey. In 18 or 20 days more we hope to land in the settlement.

Monday 13th. Morning appears lowery[51] [then] partialy clears away. Started at 1/2 past 8 when a tremendious shower ensued. Company generaly got very wet. Encamped until afternoon. Travelled this day 15 miles.

Tuesday 14th. Started 7 ock. Nooned at 10. Discovered that my acid bottle had sprung a leak the stopple having got lose and had like to have ruined my trunk. But fortunately discovered it before much damage was done. At 4 ock as we were upon the eve of Starting Andrews who had been loss eight days hove in sight. He had been captivated [captured] by the Indians but fortunately made his escape in the night. Having received no harm from them, nor did they show any hostile intentions. Traveled this day 22 miles. Encamped on the river.

Wednesday 15th. High wind last night and some rain. Mr. Knight had his hat blown from his head last night & not able to find it this morning furnish him myself with one. We conclude to cross the

---

Missouri in the fall of 1822 with a caravan bound for Santa Fe. On the Arkansas winter overtook them. Their animals wandered off or died, so when spring came the traders cached their goods and went on to Taos for more animals. Returning to their caches they recovered their property and continued their journey to Santa Fe." Brown, *Santa Fe Trail*, 103; Josiah Gregg, *Commerce of the Prairies*, 47.

[50]Dr. Willard's party of packers would have camped halfway between present-day Cimarron and Ingalls, Kansas.

[51]"Lowery" or "loury" is another word for a gloomy, cloudy sky.

river[52] at this place and lay in our meat for the remaining part of the journey. Went out with three others to kill meat. Shot and brot in two which we *jourked* or dried. Made 2 skin tubs which we crossed all the goods in with perfect safety and those of us that could not swim. Andrews meets with another accident. While attempting to cross the river on a mule got entangled in some way and to save his life threw his rifle which he had swam the rivers twice before with by the aid of a billet of wood carying it on his back. He made several trials to hook it up without success.

Thursday 16th. Weather fine. Spend the day in manufacturing our provisions.

Friday 17th. Morning pleasant. Stood a volunteer gard last night. Heavy dew and musquetoes troublesome. Captain wrote a letter put it under a B. Skin. [He] put up a guide board pointing to it expecting the waggoners would find it. Buffalo and like most of the waters of this country is slightly impregnated with some mineral.

Monday 20th. Started at 5. Nooned at 1/2 past 10. Buffalo more plenty killed 5 or 6 this day. Frequently see wild horses but cant approach them. Sultry and Sandy, traveling tedious. Usual course of river S.W. Travelled this day 24 miles. Encamped without wood. Buffalo dung is the only fuel to be obtained on this river.

Tuesday 21st. Stood extra guard last night. Mr. Glass had a severe turn of the colic which required my attention several hours. Started

---

[52]The group of packers crossed the Arkansas River at the Upper Crossing, east of Lakin, Kansas. Throughout the 1820s the Upper Crossing of the Arkansas River was the most frequently used crossing by Santa Fe Trail traders because of its rocky riverbed. When Willard's group used this crossing, Captain McKnight left mail for the wagons following the same route. On September 26, 1825, the Sibley survey party also used this crossing. They then traveled westward along the south side of the river, noting Indian Mound and Chouteau's Island, before traveling south to the Sand Hills following Bear Creek through Bear Creek Pass. In 1829 the trade caravan, accompanied by the first military escort on the Santa Fe Trail, also crossed here. For years trail scholars have relied on Josiah Gregg's 1844 account that the Middle Crossing served as the main route over the Arkansas River, which was the international boundary with Mexico. Dr. Willard's account, along with George C. Sibley's 1825 journal and diary and subsequent trade caravans, officially establish the Upper Crossing as the preferred trail route throughout the 1820s. In fact, the Upper Crossing was easier for wagons than the Middle Crossing, because the banks were not steep and the riverbed was rocky rather than sandy.

at 5. Turned out at 10. Wind more brisk and travelling better. Passed 2 or 3 springs. Killed 5 or 6 Buffalo. Started again at 4—Mare ran away. Lost one of my pistols which gave me a considerable trouble in finding it. Encamped at 7. Travelled this day 25 miles, grass getting better and Buffalo become Scarcer.

Wednesday 22d. Started at 1/2 past five. Travelled 5 hours and refreshed. Since we left the Arkansas we start as soon as we can hitch up after daylight generally traveling 15 miles before breakfast. Travelled this day 24 miles.

Thursday 23d. Morning fair and cool. Started at 5. Turned out at 8 by a fine Spring[53] which is surrounded by huge rocky nobs on the top of one are fortifications of rock thrown up on the verge of the eminence evidently the work [of] Indians. The borders of this spring are thickly skirted with small timber, wild plumbs, grapes, currents, &c. This variety afforded much pleasure, after being so long confine to the same expanse of Prairie. The sweet fragrance that arrose from the various blossoms, and the singing of the birds aforded singular charms. Left the Simi Rone[54] this morning and lay our course for the mountains in a south west diretion. Found plenty of water in the prairie. Traveled this day 20 miles.[55]

Friday 24. Started at 1/4 of 6. Came to a fine spring at 1/2 past 9 [and] turned out. It was reported by two of the hunters that they saw at a distance 100 head of mules and horses traveling north East and drove by Spaniard or Indians (the Spring Co. going into Missouri). Caught up at 2 but did not start consequent to an approaching shower which went mostly arround but concluded to turn out and stay until morning.

---

[53]Also known as Upper Spring, Flag Spring earned its name from a guide flag mounted on a high crag by a trader at some earlier time. Brown, *Santa Fe Trail;* Franzwa, *Maps,* 128–29. George Sibley wrote in his journal on Friday, October 7, 1825: "Situated amidst huge rocky cliffs The Upper Semerone [Cimarron] Spring, affording abudance of excellent Water, and the long narrow Valley that it waters supplied us with plenty of Wood for fuel & pretty good pasturage for our horses. This is a noted camping place, and is the point from whence we are to take our departure across a sort of Sandy desart [*sic*] to another Creek to the West." Kate Gregg, *Road to Santa Fe,* 93.
[54]Numerous trail travelers misspelled the Cimarron River.
[55]Willard's party would have passed Cold Spring, where they found plenty of water in the prairie. Their camp was about 4 miles west of Cold Spring.

Turned very cold at night with heavy dew. The country on our right presents a more broken appearance skirted with small cedar timbers.[56]

Saturday 25. Started at 1/4 past 7. Lay our course for the rabit Ears.[57] Two adjacent knobs by that name. Saw a few Buffalo today. Came to a pond of water at 1/2 past eleven. Encamped at night on the R. Ear creek.[58] Found a plenty of wood. Prairies more rolling. Traveled this day 20 miles.

Sunday 26th. Morning fine and cool. Started 1/4 past 6 direction S.W. The Rocky Mountains begin to heave in Sight. A portentious cloud gathered over us threatening hail, but fortunately went mostly arround. Traveled this day 25 miles. Encamped by a pond of water without wood. Used B. [buffalo] dung which we gathered and covered before the rain.

Monday 27. Started 1/4 past 6. Morning fine and cool. A heavy shower arrose at 2 when we were obliged to encamp without wood. Gathered dung but unable to make it burn without the assistance of old clothes & plenty of tallow, through which means we were able to boil a kettle of coffee and dry our clothes a little. This night was cold and unpleasant. Traveled 15 ms.

Friday [Tuesday] 28th. Morning cool but pleasant. Started 1/4 after 5. Found timber at 9 when we made a halt. Caught up again at eleven. Heavy Shower at 3 with some hail. Encamped on the side of a cedar ridge having found the Spanish trail. Traveled 25 miles.[59]

---

[56] This location is very likely Cedar Spring. Franzwa, *Maps*, 61.

[57] Rabbit Ears was a landmark along the Cimarron route. It was the focal point for a series of camps and trail landmarks that includes McNees Crossing, Turkey Creek Camp, Rabbit Ears Creek Camp, and Round Mound as a westbound traveler approached present-day Clayton, New Mexico. Brown, *Santa Fe Trail*, 126.

[58] Willard is mistaken. This site would be Turkey Creek Camp opposite Rabbit Ears Mountain. "At Rabbit Ears Creek (like other 'creeks' in this country dry except for the springs in its bed) fine meadows and constant water beckoned the traders to rest. Often they laid over here a day to refresh the animals." Ibid., 28–29.

[59] Their 9 A.M. halt was probably Point of Rocks, where there were springs. Today's Black Jack and Youngblood Canyons probably contained trees, based on the prominent ridges with cedars on them. Later, on October 18, 1825, George Sibley describes finding in the vicinity of Point of Rocks "a very plain Trace which leads directly to the Pass of the Mountains by which mules usually enter the Valley of Taos." Ibid., 131–34.

Wednesday 29th. Morning fine. Heavy showers last night. Stood gard this morning. We are now in sight of mountains that are perfectly white envelloped in snow. This is certainly a novel specticle. It is reputably said that they are 100 miles distant. This may be said to be an anomalous climate. Started at 9. Came to a creek 9 miles distant said to be a tributary of the Red River.[60] Here a shower insued with heavy thunder and lightning. Alternate showers all day and night. Obliged to lay in wet clothes and blankets. This was a disagreable night. After getting a little warm was called up from supposition that Indians were lurking arround us. Put my weapons in readyness & lay down. Shortly after was again alarmed by the news of about 1/4 of the horses being gone. This was painful news to the owners. But one of the company feeling unwilling to believe the Indians had taken them followed down the creek a short distance where he found them. It appeared that the first gard neglected to drive them all up it being somewhat dark when they were herded. Started this day at 1/4 of 5 and performed 30 miles.

Friday 1st July. Encamped last night half way up the mountains. Fine grass wood & water. Heavy showers last night. Started last morning at 6. Passed several snowbanks this day. Road exceedingly steep and rocky.[61] Traveled this day 25 miles. Encamped in 12 mile of TauSe [Taos]. The atmosphere on the mountain feels like the month of march. Strawberries and other vegetation in a blossom. Everything exhibits the opening of spring.

Saturday 2d. Morning fine. Stood gard last night. Every man buisy this morning in shifting clothes and washing off[62] some of the grease which has become almost indelible. Started this morning at 6. Meet 10 or a dozen Spaniards 3 miles from town who came to meet us to

---

[60]This is the Canadian River, often mistaken as a tributary of the Red River.

[61]Willard likely went west from present-day Rayado, New Mexico, following the Taos Trail, then crossed over the divide using Apache Pass and descending down into Valle Escondido, twelve miles from Taos, New Mexico.

[62]One trail into Taos followed the Río Fernando from Valle Escondido into Taos Valley. Since the men were "washing up" it would appear they were on the Río Fernando. The Sangre de Cristo Mountains east of Taos Valley were an almost impassable barrier to the eastern plains of New Mexico. Pack trains could cross over the mountains, but wagons had to follow the trail across the eastern plains of New Mexico on to Santa Fe. Hawk, "Camino Antiguos," chapter 3.

prevent our smugling or hiding goods in the mountains. All goods were taken into custody except my own, which I was permitted to take and was conducted to the house of the Alkalde[63] where I meet with a friendly reception. but on being informed that my effects were not altogether safe at his hand he having stood in the Pillory for the crime of Stealing left his house the next day which is always considered an insult to by Spaniards.

Commenced bourding **Sunday 3d July** with Pablo Luceero[64] at $12 pr month at which place I feel perfectly saf it having the name of the best house in town. Had 2 calls for medical aid. Appears to be but little regard to religion here. They have a mud church of considerable magnitude. A short service today. The Priest employed most of the day in doing business for the company. Several Fangdangoes[65] in afternoon & evening. Manners extremely rude and uncouth. Ladies tawney and void of beauty or modesty. Commenced giving Mr. Carrel[66] medicine today.

Monday 4th. This is an anniversary ever dear to an American. Am determined to commemorate it in some way. Persuade the company to go through & on firing evolutions.[67] I also prepared a flag on which I

---

[63]The correct spelling is "alcalde." The alcalde held the highest municipal position, with some duties that correspond to modern mayors, judges, and city councilors. Sometime after June 8, 1825, Pedro Martínez was temporarily serving as the constitutional alcalde of Taos with Pablo Lucero and Blas Trujillo as his assistants. Severino Martínez (the father of Padre Martínez) had served as constitutional alcalde earlier in 1825 and would again resume those duties by December 1825 and continuing into 1826. Correspondence, Spanish Archives of New Mexico (SANM I), Microfilm Roll 9 of the translations, Record 1297.

[64]In June 1825 Pablo Lucero witnessed a water document for the constitutional alcalde, Pedro Martínez. Ibid. Lucero (1782–?) was the son of Salvador Manuel Lucero de Godoy and Maria Manuela Vallejos. He was married to Maria Paula Larranaga and they had six children. He served as alcalde of Taos on numerous occasions. In 1815 he was ordered by the governor, Albero Maynex, to grant Severino Martínez (the father of Padre Antonio José Martínez) farming land on San Cristobal Creek. Ibid.; Weber, *Edge of Empire*, 26; 1850 Federal Census, ancestry.com (accessed October 21, 2009).

[65]A fandango is a popular dance somewhat similar to, or at least culturally equivalent to, what many know as a social or barn dance. Some were part of political festivities such as the Fourth of July; others played a part in religious festivities such as Christmas, and still others were held to celebrate the arrival of travelers.

[66]Febeanes Carel is listed as a trader who went to the customhouse in Santa Fe on July 9 with a factura from Columbia, dated April 26. Weber, *Extranjeros*, 17.

[67]An evolution is a military procedure broken down into individual steps to form a pattern produced by a series of repeated movements. A common example includes the steps that need to be taken to clean, load, prime, and fire a musket.

placed the resemblance of the American Eagle to show to the natives our national pride and glory. Several Fandangoes all night. Our fireing brot many citizens to witness the novel scene. After the military evolutions were through a procession of Citizens & Americans was formed with music at the head and marched to every part of the town under loud exclamations of *Viva La Republica*. The recreation of the day was claded[68] by two crowded Fangdangoes, where every American was invited. This was somewhat novel to the Americans to see the singularity of dress manners and stile and manouvres in conducting the dance. The Priest,[69] Alcalde[70] & first caracters of the place were present.[71]

Tuesday 5th. Imploy most of this day in reading and writing and feel much relieved from the fatigue of a journey. Ate some chile in the evening which made me quite ill for a few hours.

Wednesday 6th. Bleed[72] Mr. Storrs[73] & a Frenchman, gave medicine

---

[68]"Claded" would seem to mean dressed, therefore Dr. Willard described the day as dressed or distinguished by two fandangos.

[69]It is uncertain which priest is being referenced. Antonio José Martínez appears to have been the *cura encargado*, or pastor in charge of both Abiquiu and Taos, in 1825. Yet Martínez doesn't become the *cura propio*, or irremovable pastor, of Taos until July 23, 1826, when he succeeds Father José Mariano Sanchez Vergara. Chávez, *But Time and Chance*, 24–27.

[70]Don Severino Martínez (1761–1827) was the elected alcalde of Taos in 1825. Born in Abiquiu, he moved his family to the Taos Valley in 1804. He learned to read and write and became a leading citizen. His son was Padre Antonio José Martínez, whom Dr. Willard refers to as the priest. Martínez and Rafael Luna, the border guard, were empowered to intercept Americans and examine their invoices and merchandise; it seems to have been customary at this time to send to Santa Fe for the customs collector, Juan Vigil, to come to Taos for the final assessment. Weber, *Taos Trappers*, 93. See also Minge, "Last Will and Testament of Don Severino Martínez," 33–56.

[71]This 1825 entry is the first known written account of an American celebration on the Fourth of July in Taos, in what would become the state of New Mexico.

[72]Bloodletting enjoyed popularity throughout the colonial period and was a panacea for all illnesses. Its use increased considerably in the early nineteenth century. Rothstein, *American Physicians in the Nineteenth Century*, 46, 50. "From the 1790's to about the middle of the 1800's was essentially the age of Heroic medicine (allopathy), and a few allopathic physicians in the United States dominated medical philosophy and education. To practice allopathic medicine, a doctor needed only a sharp lancet to slice into a vein or leeches to suck blood from his patient, suction cups to enhance blood flow from small incisions or to withdraw 'toxins' from an inflamed part of the body, ipecac to produce vomiting, calomel to empty the bowels, and mustard to make a plaster to burn blisters on the skin. These ancient therapies were based on the premise that toxins could be extracted from a sick body via bodily fluids. Even after allopathy began to lose it luster, many frontier doctors still insisted that clysters (enemas), cathartics, and sometime cupping were the answer to most complaints." Steele, *Bleed, Blister, and Purge*, 1–3.

[73]This is probably Ricardo Storrs, a fur trapper who worked along the Colorado and *(continued)*

to another. Also obtain a case of venerial [disease]. Spent most of the day in town.

Thursday 7th. Custom House Officer arrives today. The company much agitated consequent to high duties. He however seems disposed to favor the Americans as much as possible and evade the law. The requisitions of the law is that all good shall be rated at the Chihuahua prices to which they add 25 percent and afterwards charge on that aggragate 15 percent. There were many articles of goods found to be contraband which the customhouse officer sent to St. Fee. ~~Paid the old alcalde for 3 meals of vituals and considered which man & Co fling~~

Friday 8th. Sent for this forenoon to pay duties on medicines. Went to see the C.H. Officer and learn the law. He agreed to go to my bourding house a mile distant and examine them and save me the trouble of bringing them in according to the order of the Alcade.

Saturday 9th. Nothing of importance this day. Gave L[awyer] Cave a dash of Pills yesterday & Bleed Migel Saxanago [Santiago?].

Sunday 10th. Bleed Stephen Marrs[74] and gave him medicine for the fever. Also bled my landlord and gave his lady pills. This evening Beheal[75] [Vigil] the C.H. [Custom House] Officer came to see my medicine but could not understand them. Got me to draw off the invoice and calculate the amount of duties (amt $6.50) and on finding the amt so small refused taking anything signifying that he would pay it himself.

Gila Rivers in 1826. Ricardo, along with Augustus Storrs, was issued guía (passport or trade permit) #49 on October 21, 1827, in Santa Fe. One would assume the two men are related, but no evidence was found to prove this conjecture. In 1828 Ricardo Storrs exported 566 pounds of furs to Saint Louis, which amounted to $4.50 per pound or $2,547 total—approximately $64,000 in today's currency. Weber, *Taos Trappers*, 134, 173; Weber, *Extranjeros*, 32.

[74]Dr. Willard's penmanship is extremely small and, coupled with his spelling, very hard to decipher. The surname is probably Marrs. A Stephan Mury [?] is listed as visiting the customhouse in Santa Fe on July 9, 1825, with a factura from Columbia, dated April 25. Weber, *Extranjeros*, 17.

[75]Juan Bautista Vigil y Alarid (1792–1866) was born in Santa Fe and married Rafaela Sánchez in Tomé in 1808. Vigil became politically active after Mexican independence and held a number of political posts, including secretary of state, in the Mexican period. He was the customhouse agent or officer from approximately 1825 to 1828. Vigil y Alarid served as a customs collector, whereby he administered trade regulations and payment of duties from merchants who brought goods from the United States along the Santa Fe Trail. Sisneros, "She Was Our Mother," 286–87; Weber, *Extranjeros*, 25. N.Mex. State Records Center and Archives, Mexican Archives of New Mexico (MANM), Jan–April 1826, Microfilm Roll 6, Frame 299.

Monday 11th. Attend to my patients in town, 1 or 2 each a day. The rest of the time imploy in reading.

Tuesday 12th. Gave Stephen Marrs Sundry medicines to take with him to St. Fee.

Wednesday 13th. Nothing of importance today Save an opperation with the Catheter on an Indian who laboured under Ischuria.[76] The opperation [was] some what difficult but succeeded. ~~in drawing his water.~~

Thursday 14th. Was visited again by my Indian patient who was again obliged to submit to another opperation with the Catheter. Also bled an old Lady and gave medicine for sore eyes. Many wanting medicine but no money to pay for it.

Friday 15th. Commenced giving medicine to Preino for a twelve years venerial [disease. He] agres to [have me] cure him for 35 dollars.

Saturday 16th. Bleed 2 Frenchmen Vausan[77] and Victor and attend to my other patients in town.

Sunday 17th. Walked to town in the morning. Spent most of the day in reading. Called on at night to visit Mr. P. Ballio[78] under fever. Stayed all night.

Monday 18th. Received a message from the priest at St. Cruise[79] wishing me to come and see his lady labouring under consumption. Started in the afternoon. Called on Mr. Ballio. Gave him a dose of physic[80] and extracted the first bone from a ladies thum. Called again at the young Priest. Gave medicine to two patients. Put up at Laureno Cordivo.[81] Bleed him and Lady well treated. Attended a Fangdango in the evening.

---

[76]Ischuria is defined as retention or suppression of urine.

[77]Jean Vaillant had arrived in New Mexico in 1824. Weber, *Taos Trappers*, 142.

[78]This is Paul Baillo, who went out to meet Sibley's survey party later in 1825 and led them across the pass into Taos Valley. Baillo had worked with George Sibley and Lilburn Boggs in the Indian trade at Fort Osage, but by 1826 he was partnered with Ceran St. Vrain to outfit trappers. Lavender, *Bent's Fort*, 374.

[79]Santa Cruz de la Cañada was located immediately east of present-day Española, New Mexico.

[80]A homeopathic drug ingested to purge the patient. It is also a cathartic, laxative, and diuretic.

[81]Lorenzo Cordova.

Tuesday 19th. Visited an old Lady this morning and Start for Santa Cruse. Reached the Priests at 1/2 past 9. Distance 50 miles and rugged mountains to cross. Felt extremely unwell in the evening from sour stomach.

Wednesday 20th. Priest absent last night returns this morning. Saw his woman who is unable to speak loud and much afflicted with a bad cough, and from a history of her case was labouring under the Phthisis Pulmunalis.[82] Gave her medicine.

Thursday 21st. Patient some better. Make preparations to return but unable to find the horse and conclude to stay until morning.

Friday 22d. Started for Tause a little after sunrise. Called at an Indian village to see the priest who was not up but was treated with a plate of cheese and a tankard of wine. Called again in another little town at the alkades house. Gave him physic, pressed me to stay all day— was called from there to see a neighboring woman labouring under Rheumatism. Bleed and gave her physic. Made several other calls on the way. Arrived at Cordivos a little after ten ock. Much fatigued and quite unwell. Retired without supper.

Saturday 23d. Arrived this morning before breakfast at my bourding house. Saw all my patients which I found doing well. Had an attact of collic in the evening, but soon got relief.

Sunday 24th. Remained at home this day and attended class to my Books. Let Mr. Chambers[83] have physic for Indian.

---

[82]Consumption of the lungs; strictly applied to the tuberculous variety. Phthisis is an archaic name for tuberculosis. Rudy's List of Archaic Medical Terms, http://www.antiquusmorbus .com/English/EnglishP.htm (accessed November 8, 2009).

[83]Samuel Chambers (1788–1860), who had been born in Virginia, was residing in Taos when Dr. Willard arrived. Weber calls Chambers a "curious and obscure figure" who joined the 1812 expedition to Santa Fe with Robert McKnight. In 1820 he was allowed to return to the United States. He went to Taos, where he was a partner in a distillery by the winter of 1824–25. Chambers remained there as a trader; he was given a guía for Santa Fe on December 20, 1827. He was still traveling the Chihuahua Trail in October 1835 as evidenced by a surviving guía. He eventually returned to Saint Louis where he resided until his death. He was married to Elizabeth Chambers and they had six children. Book of Guías for Santa Fe/1826–1828; Weber, *Taos Trappers*, 60, 72–73, 115, 118; Josiah Gregg, *Commerce of the Prairies*, 5–7, 56; Weber, *Extranjeros*, 33; 1850 United States Federal Census, ancestry.com (accessed November 11, 2013).

Monday 25. Bleed a Spaniard for Mr. Preino. This is an anniversary of St. James with the Spanish who spend the day in recreations.

Tuesday 26th. Start this morning to visit some of the little villages below. Received a polite invitation to attend a Fandango this eve. Mr. Anderson returns home with me and persuades me to go back with him again, and start in the morning with him to visit a warm Spring 3 miles distant from his lodgings. Agree to go. Called at the Fangdango in few minutes persuaded me to dance.

Wednesday 27th. Started this morning after breakfast to visit the spring, which we found worthy our attention. The water is a little more than blood warm and of a slight brackish tast. These waters are said to have cured several cases of rheumatism & some other diseases. Mr. Walsh[84] left today. Gave him medicines to take with him. Left medicine for the alkades wife.

Thursday 28th. Nothing of importance transpires today. Save the Patch[85] [Apache] nation of Indians have retreated to this settlement for safety from the Navihos. Lucero takes my horses.

Friday 29th. My patients mostly off my hands. Dull times and no money. Received a letter yesterday from Capt. Morris at Santa Fe[86] with the compliments of the Govr. and the Priest at the St. Cruis wishing me to visit them. Mr. Rubedois'[87] company started on Wednesday last for Missouri. Being absent, neglected to write by them. Sent for

---

[84]Unknown trader.

[85]Presumed to be Jicarilla Apache.

[86]Governor Pedro de Peralta laid out the plan for the new Villa de Santa Fé by the spring of 1610. Hordes, "History of Santa Fe Plaza," 132. The Spanish colonial census of 1790 for Santa Fe listed 2,396 residents.

[87]Dr. Willard states that Robidoux's company left Taos on July 27, 1825. "On August 30, 1825, *'Robideaus party from Tous'* returned to the Council Bluffs. These fur returns may have been brought in by François or Louis Robidoux." Barry, *Beginning of the West,* 118. Francisco Ruidu [Robidoux], Miguel Rubidu, and Antonio Rubidu are all declared merchants and without passports in the February 1826 Report on Foreigners written by Governor Antonio Narbona. These reports were mandated after a circular dated November 19, 1825, ordered each Mexican state and territory to make a monthly report of the number and movement of all foreigners to the Secretaría de Relaciones Interiores y Exteriores. Weber, *Extranjeros,* 19–22.

this evening to visit Sr. Lunas[88] labouring under plurisy.[89] At the same time visited the Alcade Lady.

Saturday 30th. Visited my patients as yesterday. Mr. Baillio's hunters have returned after 90 miles travel for fear of Indian depredations, having been followed by them several days. They start again today a different course. This company was robbed of 17 horses the first evening after they started, but sent back and got more. They are determined however to persevere but are obliged to git licenses for trapping within this Territory. Felt indisposed this evening from colic pains consequent to eating S[our] Cheese.

Sunday 31st. Health very good this morning though was quite ill untill after midnight. Weather quite sultry and the earth very much parched there having been no rain (save a few Sprinkles twice) for more than a month. Went to town in the afternoon. Was called to two places, one to a woman who was taken speachless and remained so 24 hours before I saw her. Was almost astonished on entering the house to find it thronged with men, women & children in so much that I was unable to approach her. She was held by her husband and suffecating for breath. This was a scene of superstition. They had got a small bell which they rang constantly together with incesant prayers. I told my interpreter to order this house cleared of the throng and to give her air. Believeing her to be somewhat spasmodic, I immediately bled her. My interpreter informed me that inquiry was made if there were no women present under ~~her course~~ as they will not suffer a woman of that discription to remain in presence of the sick. They are also particular in the choice of a bandage for the area where bled, cautiously avoiding (~~the lower portion of women's shirt~~) certain things. Before I left town an Indian Chief called on me labouring under the dropsy.[90]

---

[88]Rafael Luna was deputized as a border guard in the spring of 1825 by the customs officer Juan Bautista Vigil y Alarid. Vigil ordered Severino Martínez and Rafael Luna to use militia to intercept American traders. Weber, *Edge of Empire*, 60, 62.

[89]Pleurisy is defined as "inflamation of the lining of the thorax, often with an effusion (collection of fluid). A common complication of pneumonia." Steele, *Bleed*, 326.

[90]Dropsy is an old term for the abnormal swelling of soft tissue due to the accumulation of excess water. Today, the description would be more specific, i.e., edema due to congestive heart failure.

Took him home with me and gave him medicine. Pulled a tooth for another Indian when I returned.

Monday 1st Augt. Another month had passed away and from $170 practice have received but 26 dollars though the majority of charges are good. Visited my patients in town [and] found them better, my Speachless patient able to talk fluently. Was sent for this afternoon to a man who had fallen from his horse and at the same time recieved a kick in the breast. Bled him &c. Was informed in the evening by my Landlord who returned from the prairie that my horses had left his gang and gone to some American herd.

Tuesday 2d. Sent a boy for my horses this morning who returned with then in the evening. Was visited by a man from St. Cruise 50 miles distant labouring under a protracted case of the stricture or gravel.[91] Took considerable pains to learn his complaint and on inquirey found he had nothing to pay [and] accordingly dismissed him. Was attacked in the night with a violent ear ache which lasted 5–6 hours and left me.

Wednesday 3d. Bleed 2 men in town. Gave one an Emetic[92] to take tomorrow morning. A considerable shower fel yesterday for this country though but barely laid the dust.

Thursday 4th. Called on to visit a patient in town before breakfast. Found him severely exercised with medicine, but doing well. Visited Mr. Rennison[93] 4 miles below [and] found him convelesent. ~~Made a~~

---

[91]*gravel:* A kidney stone (renal calculus) forms in the kidney from substances that would normally pass out of the body in the urine. When there are large amounts of these substances, they separate from the urine and form kidney stones.

[92]An emetic, or drug that causes vomiting such as syrup of ipecac, has unpredictable effects, often causing prolonged vomiting.

[93]John Rennison (1779–1844) was born in England. He married Jane Creighton on May 13, 1799, at Saint Mary's Church in Carlisle, Cumberland County, England. He was a tailor by occupation. In Carlisle living conditions were so bad in 1812 that hunger riots occurred. In 1819 the weavers of Carlisle petitioned the prince regent to be sent to America to escape the terrible conditions in which they lived and worked. In August 1820 John and Jane Rennison and their family arrived at Philadelphia from Liverpool, England, aboard the *Liverpool Packet*. The Rennisons eventually traveled to Missouri, where John patented land in Cooper County, Missouri. He is listed on July 8 in the Santa Fe customhouse records for 1825 with a factura from Franklin, April 30. Weber, *Extranjeros*, 17. He died in Cooper County, Missouri, in 1844 without leaving a will. "John Rennison," http://familytreemaker.genealogy.com/users/c/o/p/Julie-A-Copple-hamilton/WEBSITE-0001/UHP-0053.html (accessed November 9, 2013).

~~proposition to take my mare to Missouri . Keep her and to breed and give me the mare and half the colts when I return or send for them. I agree to his proposition.~~

Friday 5th. Spend this day in reading. A light shower today.

Saturday 6th. Nothing of consequence transpires today. Remain at home it being a pleasant retreat.

Sunday 7th. A few shower to day which is very unusual in this country at this time of year. Rode to town where I found it in complete confusion it being made a day of Sport then was dancing rasing ever lasting whopping and holloring as is the practice of this country.

Monday 8th. Called on early this morning by the Alcade to visit his Lady.[94] Did so. Attended a fangdango in the evening from special invitations. Little satisfaction to be realized amongst them.

Tuesday 9th. Mr. Rennison came to stay with me a while being in delicate health.

Wednesday 10th. Visited the Indian Chief of the [Taos] tribe.[95] Find him very ill of the dropsy. Expressed abundant gratitude for my compliment by setting me the best that his house could afford consisting of soup, meat, flour bread, corn cakes, raspberries, ~~and~~ black currands, &c. and pressed me to take with me when I left.

Thursday 11th. Nothing transpires today of importance. Rode to the distillery for Spts[96] of wine.

Friday 12th. Visited Severino this morning. Found the old Lady better. Called at Sr. Lunas. Opened his servt. girl's thum [and] ordered a

---

[94]Maria del Carmel Santistevan was married to Don Severino Martínez in 1787 at the village of Santo Tomas de Abiquiu. She and her husband had six children, the eldest of which was the priest Don Antonio José Martínez. Archives of Archdiocese of Santa Fe, Reel 26, Abiquiu Marriages 1777–1826, Frame 850.

[95]Willard uses the term "Chief" in its generic sense, as was usually the case with Anglo writers describing native social structures in the nineteenth century. Willard, like most foreigners, would likely not have known of the Spanish form of secular government that had existed at Taos Pueblo since the seventeenth century, with its annual nomination process, the election of a governor and other officers, and its array of administrative officials. M. Estellie Smith, *Governing at Taos Pueblo* ([Portales]: Paleo-Indian Institute, Eastern New Mexico University, 1969), 10–26.

[96]Spirits of wine, meaning brandy. Samuel Chambers, James Baird, Thomas Long, "Peg-leg" Smith, and a man named Stevens built the first distillery in Taos. Weber, *Taos Trappers*, 72, 118. See also Weber, "William Workman," 155–61.

salve made. Afternoon visited the Pueblo villiage. Called on my Indian patient [and] found him ill. Glad to see me. Me and my company conclude to visit the Cathc priest, who we found in fine humour. Had much conversation on different subjects such as geography, politicks, &c. Urged us to stay all night & would not take no for an answer until I urged the necessity of visiting a patient that evening when he consented.

Saturday 13th. Went to town this morning [and] found several of my Missouri friends. Wrote 2 letters in the afternoon to my friends in Missouri.

Sunday 14th. Sent for early this morning to visit a man at the Ranch[os de Taos] who has a Polypus[97] in the nose and a Polypus or fungus excrescence[98] in the eye ~~and~~ of an enourmous size. He begs me to excise the excrescence feeling willing to run all risks trusting in his God. Agree to visit him again. Gave medicine to a young Lady for slight spasms in the Stomach and returned home. Was called on in the evening to visit a man afflected with Phymosis.[99] Unable to pay me, bleed and give him medicine.

Monday 15. Sent for to visit young Cordiva under fever and a lance arm from Bleding. Staid all night better in the morning.

Tuesday 16. Returned from Sr. Cordivas this morning on foot. After-noon visited my patients at the Ranch with Mr. Baillio. Came by Cordivas house. On my return found the family Considerably agitated from a near encampment of Indians.

Wednesday 17. Visited a woman in town labouring under the Pleurisy. Also visited my patient with a lance arm and found they had neglected him arm highly inflamed and some fever. Gave him a dose of Salts[100] [and] returned home.

Thursday 18th. Showers on the mountains for several days past. The air feels like the fall of the year. Visited Cordivo today.

---

[97]Polypus is another word for polyp.

[98]An excrescence could be a growth, wart, or tumor that is either useless or disfiguring.

[99]Phimosis is an abnormal constriction of the foreskin that prevents it from being drawn back to uncover the glans penis. "Rudy's List of Archaic Medical Terms," www.antiguusmorbus.com (accessed September 22, 2012).

[100]Epsom salts to relieve inflammation.

Friday 19th. Visited Cordivo [and] found him much better the inflamation having considerably abated.

Saturday 20. Visited Cordivo. Attended a Fangdango in the evening at Sr. Lunars. Retired early. The manners and costoms seem to improve a little.

Sunday 21st. Visited my sick patient at the Ranch[101] and performed an opperation on his eye by extracting the same. This was a painful task, the eye being obliterated in a great measure, and the socket filled with a morbid excrescence forming a very considerable protubercule and firmly based upon the bone in and about the socket. Left him considerably exhausted. Felt samething indisposed from a slight fever after my return home.

Monday 22d. Visited my patient at the Ranch. Found him quite comfortable. Heavy showers in afternoon with considerable hail.

Tuesday 23?[102] Visited my patient at the Ranch.

Wednesday 24th. Visited Cordivo & my man at the Ranch, got caught in a heavy shower.

Thursday 25. Visited the Ranch in the afternoon. The Americans begin to collect in order to [get] organized for their departure.

Friday 26. Visited Cordivo by the Ranch—find him nearly well.

Saturday 27. Visited the Ranch by Cordivo in company with an interpreter. Sold my necklace for a Dispusaton. Gave a fangdango in the evening.

Sunday 28. Spent most of the day in writing letters.

Monday 29. Visited the Ranch [and] found Capt. Means[103] & some other Americans.

---

[101]Modern usage would tend to suggest that the "Ranch" would refer to Rancho de Taos, but it is not clear that such generalized usage was common in the early 1800s.

[102]The question mark is Willard's notation. He apparently was uncertain of the date.

[103]John Means presented a factura listed as #24 in December 1826 when he paid duties to the customhouse officer. Weber, *Extranjeros*, 27.

Tuesday 30th. Purchased cloathes of Clapton.[104] Attended a Fang-dango in the evening at Mr. Beards.[105]

Wednesday 31st. Visited the Ranch by Cordivos. My friends advise me to remain in this part of the country a year longer before I go below in order to git the language and having seen a letter from Sonora stating the scarcity of medicine conclude to stay on another year in order to obtain medicine from Missouri and accordingly send on a bill to that effect.

Thursday 1st. September. Mr. Rennison came to stay with me last night. He proposes sending me a suit of clothes next season. I agree to go and encamp with the company who start today for Missouri. Made fifteen miles when we overtook a part of the company that started yesterday. A light shower in the evening.

Friday 2d. Night cool. Mr. Cave was quite sick last night with fever. Bled him. Better this morning. Was requested to assist in enroll-ing and organizing the [eastbound] company. Elected R. W. Morris Captain [and] divided them into 17 messes, there being 75 or 80 in all. It is supposed they have 700 head of horses & mules.[106] Parted with company after breakfast and returned much fatigued.

---

[104]Unknown trader.

[105]James Baird (1767–1826) was born in Pennsylvania and died in Ciudad Juárez. He traveled west from Pennsylvania and set up a general store in Saint Louis in 1810. In 1812 Baird joined Robert McKnight, Samuel Chambers, and others to form a trading company that traveled to Taos, where they were arrested. First they were sent to Santa Fe and then on to Chihuahua, where they were detained for nearly a decade. After his release in 1820, Baird returned to Saint Louis. In 1822 Baird led a small company of six men across the plains to Santa Fe. This time they hit the jackpot. In 1825 he was among the group that established the first distillery near Taos, New Mexico. Baird became a Mexican citizen and settled at El Paso del Norte, where in 1826 he protested to his government against the inroads being made by Americans on the Mexican beaver-trapping business. Subsequently Baird, who lived in and around Chihuahua, also worked as a trapper in the Gila region of today's New Mexico, where he died. He was buried in Ciudad Juárez. A number of Americans were included as *albaceas*, or witnesses to his probate. Josiah Gregg, *Commerce of the Prairies*, 12.

[106]For the year 1825, Josiah Gregg estimates the Santa Fe merchandise trade valued at $65,000 with 130 men. Willard's diary entry is corroborated by the *Missouri Republican* in an account dated October 24, 1825. Archibald Gamble, the secretary for the Sibley survey of the road to Santa Fe, states, "The expedition reached the boundary line early in Sept. and remained in camp until the 21st, waiting for the authority to continue the surveys through the Mexican territory." The commissioners were Major Sibley, Colonel Reeves, and Colonel Mather. *(continued)*

Saturday 3d. Visited the Ranch. Feel something melancholy since Americans left here.

Sunday 4. Came to a determination to leave this place and spend the winter and spring at the pass.[107]

Monday 5th. Begin to settle my business and prepared for a start.

Tuesday 6th. Settled with my landlord allow him 12 dollars a month for board. Visited the Ranch afternoon.

Wednesday 7. Spend most of my time in reading.

Thursday 8. Nothing of importance.

Friday 9. Called on to visit a woman in town afflicted with a pain in her face and says she has discharged large amount from her nose with some fever.

Saturday 10. Visited Ranch. Treated 2 new patients, one with fever, the other Rheumatism. Occupied from the 10 to the 15th in preparing to start to the Pass but have had but little success in collecting.

Friday 15.[108] Started from Taos. Traveled 18 miles. Called at Cordivos in the morning for money due me [but] refused to pay. Cussed and quit him.

Saturday 16th. Started at day brake. Called at John Andrews.[109] Bled

---

At North Bend, on the return, "a company of 20 adventurers with a great many mules and horses laden with merchandize, arrived from Missouri, bound for Santa Fe; and an hour afterwards a company of 81 persons, returning from Santa Fe, also arrived at their camp." This company carried:

In Silver,	$18,568
Gold	182
Beaver Fur, 2,044 @ $5	$10,220
Mules 416, Jacks and Jennets 25, Horses 189 = 630 @ $25 =	$15,700
	Total of $44,670.

Barry, *Beginning of the West*, 126; Josiah Gregg, *Commerce of the Prairies*, 332.

[107]He is referring to El Paso del Norte, which today is Ciudad Juárez.

[108]Dr. Willard's dates are in error here and not in synchronization. He straightens out the days and dates on Tuesday the 20th.

[109]Later in the diary a John Anderson from Santa Cruz arrives in Chihuahua on November 21, 1825. I believe John Andrews and John Anderson are one and the same, although I'm uncertain which last name is correct.

and gave him physic. Called at Priest Rados[110] who appeared glad to see us. Reached St. Fee at sunset. Put up with Sr. Vigill who treated me well.

Sunday 17. This place contain about 2,000 Inhabitants the major part of them quite poor and the country arround it entirely barren. It was founded the beginning of the 17th Century now in a State of decline. This day is cool and rainy.

Monday 18th. The mountains are white with snow this morning and the mercury stands at 50 F.H.[111] Attended a Fangdango in the evening given by the Americans.

Tuesday 20. Treated Sr. Vigills Lady for an accute Rheumatism [and] was very successful in relieving her. Called on today to visit the Govr.[112] Found him slightly indisposed. Gave him a dose of Physic and several visits. Attended another Fandango at night.

---

[110]This is Manuel de Jesús Rada (1788–1843) who was born in Durango, Mexico. He died and was buried in Parral, Mexico. Rada, a priest, arrived in New Mexico in 1821 after he was appointed by the bishop of Durango to fill the vacant benefice in the parish of Santa Cruz de la Cañada in New Mexico. He served there *en propiedad*, that is, with the expectation that he would derive his livelihood from the post. He served until his election by the voters of New Mexico Territory to represent them at the national congress in Mexico City in October 1828. Rada also served as pastor at San Juan Pueblo (1826–28) and as vicar for the Río Arriba parishes (1826–28). Today, San Juan Pueblo is called by its Tewa name of Ohkay Owingeh. Weber, *Northern Mexico*, 17–18; Hendricks, "Father Manuel Rada," 9–17, 24.

[111]Fahrenheit.

[112]Antonio Narbona (1773–1830) was born at Mobile in Spanish Louisiana, now Alabama. He was a *criollo*, or locally born person of pure Spanish ancestry. He arrived in Sonora in 1789 as a cadet in the Santa Cruz Company, sponsored by the commandant, Brigadier Enrique Grimarest, who was his brother-in-law. He was promoted to ensign of the Fronteras garrison in Sonora on January 27, 1793. Lieutenant Antonio Narbona came to New Mexico from Chihuahua province in January 1805 as the head of a unit of soldiers sent to respond to a Navajo raid. From 1809 to 1825 he continued his military career in Sonora and Sinoloa, where he was promoted in 1825. Colonel Antonio Narbona was appointed *géfe político* (equivalent to governor) of New Mexico from September 1825 to May 1827. In 1825 the U.S. president James Monroe sent three representatives to Santa Fe, New Mexico, to negotiate a "road between nations" and to establish trade routes and define hunting rights. George Sibley met with Governor Narbona and established cordial relations. As governor, he issued beaver-trapping licenses to foreigners from the United States on condition that they took Mexicans with them and taught them the skills. However, in 1826 he sent a report to the national government in which he expressed concern about the number of Anglo-Americans who had moved into Taos and Santa Fe. These did not just include merchants but also tradesmen such as carpenters, smiths, cabinet makers, painters, and even hat makers. He died in Arizpe, Sonora, on March 20, 1830. "Antonio Narbona," http://en.wikipedia.org/wiki/Antonio_Narbona (last modified on June 4, 2014).

Wednesday 21st. Visited the Governor. Found him in tolerable health though with a slight pain in the head and some fever. Bled him and gave him Crm. Tart.[113] Also opened an absess on his daughter's knee. The Governor expresses much intrest in my behalf and presents me with a first rate mule. Likewise he offers giving me letters to the first men in Chauaua [Chihuahua] &c.

Thursday 22d. Weather cool. Visited the Governor [and] found him restored to health. Daughter succeeding fast. Pay her a visit 2 or 3 times a day.

Friday 23. Remains cool and snow remains on the mountain. Visit the Governor as usual.

Saturday 24th. Weather more pleasant. Fangdango tonight and one last night.

Sunday 25th. Attend church this morning. Worship similar to the same denomination in Missouri. Fangdango at night.

Monday 26th. Nothing of importance transpires except the mail arrives and learns the news of a war between Russia, France & Spain against England North & Spanish America.

Tuesday 27th. Nothing of importance today save Campbell,[114] Emmons[115] & Storrs[116] leaves for the Pass.

---

[113]Cream of tartar, also known as potassium bitartrate, a common, mild laxative.

[114]Richard Campbell (?–1860) is listed on April 7, 1825, in the customhouse Records of Santa Fe. Both Richard Campbell and Ira A. Emmons were issued either guía #13 or #10 for Sonora dated September 23, 1825, under Miscellaneous Guías. Weber, *Extranjeros*, 17, 24. At one time Richard Campbell may have been considered one of the most important fur traders in the Southwest, but he remains an obscure figure today. Campbell led a group of thirty-five men from Taos to San Diego, arriving in the fall of 1827 as the first Taos trapper to reach California. He had returned to New Mexico by late February 1828. He married Maria Rosa Grijalva at Taos in September 1828 and became a Mexican citizen in 1829. He died in New Mexico in 1860, after briefly working as a miner, a sheriff, and a probate judge. Weber, *Taos Trappers*, 134–36; Weber, *Mexican Frontier*, 143.

[115]Ira A. Emmons seems to have had a reputation as an experienced trader in Santa Fe. George Sibley recommended Emmons as captain for the government's survey party in the spring of 1825. Instead, Emmons helped lead the annual summer caravan to Santa Fe and received a trade

Wednesday 28th. Expected to have started for the Pass today [but] Ward[117] not ready.

Thursday 29. All ready to start to day but our interpreter is detained for debt. Started from St. Fee at 8 ock and camped in the Canion.[118] 15 miles.

Friday 30th. Started at daylight. Cold last night. Called at St. Domingo,[119] an Indian village who appear poor & dirty.

Saturday 1st October. Encamped last night on a beautiful green by the river. Travelled 15 miles.

Sunday 2d. Stayed last night six miles above Albakirky [Albuquerque]. Came to town at 9 [and] put up at the Alcades.[120] Sold a few goods in the course of the day.

---

permit for Sonora in the fall. He is missing from documentation until April 23, 1827, when "as one of the five 'Americanos,' he showed up in Santa Fe, having 'returned to the territory from a distant land.'" Weber, *Taos Trappers*, 127–28.

[116]Augustus Storrs (1791–1850) was born on April 5, 1791, in Hanover, New Hampshire. He served as postmaster and clerk in the Missouri state legislature but was more interested in business than politics. He was on a caravan to Santa Fe as early as 1823 and later traded goods on the Santa Fe Trail. In 1825 he was appointed U.S. consul for Santa Fe, and by February 1826 he was living in El Paso del Norte. Weber, *Extranjeros*, 22; William E. Bard, "Storrs, Augustus," *Handbook of Texas Online*, http://www.tshaonline.org/handbook/online/articles/fst67 (accessed May 6, 2013); Walter B. Smith II, *America's Diplomats and Consuls*, 223.

[117]Juan Worde [John Ward] (1795–1870) was born in Ireland. As a trader he lived in Santa Fe, Chihuahua, and Parral and served as a U.S. consul to Mexico. He died in New Orleans, Louisiana. He is listed as a merchant without a passport from a report Governor Antonio Narbona created, which was "probably his first response to a circular of November 19, 1825, which ordered each Mexican state and territory to make a monthly report of a number and movement of all foreigners to the Secretaria de Relaciones Interiores y Exteriores." At the time Ward had settled in Santa Fe. Weber, *Extranjeros*, 20–21.

[118]Cañon del Río Santa Fe, south of La Cienega, New Mexico.

[119]American anthropologist Leslie White wrote in 1935 that Santo Domingo was "the most important of the Keresan pueblos." The long-standing general prestige of Santo Domingo may be attributed to a number of factors: (1) The pueblo was the ecclesiastic capital of New Mexico. The Franciscans had their headquarters there, including their archives. (2) Situated on the east side of the Río Grande, the pueblo was directly on or near the established roads, from the Camino Real or early Spanish times to the modern state and federal highways. In 1807 the pueblo held an estimated 1,000 persons. Sturtevant, Ortiz, and Lange, *Handbook of North American Indians Southwest*, 9:379–80; Jackson, *Following the Royal Road*, 34.

[120]Manuel Armijo (1795–1853) was listed as the alcalde of Albuquerque in December 1825, so presumably he was alcalde when Dr. Willard traveled through Albuquerque in early October 1825. Mexican Archives of New Mexico (MANM), Frame 918, Roll #4, 1824–1825.

Monday 3d. Conclude to stay this day for the purpose of trading.

Tuesday 4th. Sold better than $100 worth of goods yesterday. Left this morning at 8 ock. Travelled 12 or 15 miles [and] put up at Mr. Montoya a dam Rascal. Stayed overnight and next day fornoon. Bill 8 dollars. Proceeded on 6 or 8 miles and put up at a small town called Toma.[121] Treatment not very good. Waited very late for supper. Became impatient and retired without. Rained last night & and this forenoon. Weather quite cool. Some snow on the mountains.

Thursday 6th. Cold last night and this morning. Some rain and snow on the mountains. My comrades opened their goods this morning but the women hooted at the any price whatever & the old woman even refused to take Sand dollars[122] the currency of the country. For our entertainment we accordingly referred our case to the alcalde who said she might do as she pleased take it or go without anything where upon we left her unpaid. Returned back 1 1/2 miles to the farm of the late Governor[123] where we concluded to stay until the next morning. Sold some goods and traded very politely. Called on in the evening to visit a Sister of the Govr. Gave her medicine.

Friday 7th. On reloading our goods this morning missed a bundle of cloths belonging to the Mr. Floid[124] (amt 20) and a bag of bread. We

---

[121]Tomé, New Mexico. The first settler in the area was Tomé Dominguez, who had an *estancia* (large ranch) there before the Pueblo Revolt. The Dominguez family left El Paso del Norte with the balance of the refugees and did not return. In the 1740s Tomé was resettled by *genízaros* as a frontier town. Bishop Tameron visited in 1760 and remarked that it was a new town with a decent church. The bishop confirmed 402 persons. Comanche attacks in 1777 and 1778 resulted in the loss of fifty-one lives. Jackson, *Following the Royal Road*, 55–56.

[122]"Sand dollar" or "sand cast dollar" was the name given to a Mexican peso cast in Chihuahua by Ferdinand VII during the Revolutionary period (1812–21). These pieces are generally counter stamped. Reilly, "Dictionary of Numismatic names," 209.

[123]The late governor, Bartolomé Baca (1767–1834), was born in Belén, New Mexico. His million-acre ranch east of the Abo Mountains was established in 1819 through a land grant awarded by Spanish governor Facundo Melgares. His three sons worked the ranch and oversaw 40,000 head of sheep, 900 cattle, and 300 mares. It was profitable until 1833 when Navajo raids increased. He abandoned the ranch after his shepherds were killed and the livestock were stolen. Miller, "Bartolomé Baca Grant."

[124]Floid is Gentry Fuyd [Floyd] who is listed as a merchant without a passport in the Report on Foreigners by Governor Antonio Narbona dated February 1, 1826. David Weber notes that Floyd would have been a resident of Santa Fe while other foreigners on the list resided in Taos. Weber, *Extranjeros*, 20–21.

suppose them to have been stolen or to have fallen out of the waggon. Left the Governors farm at 9 Ock. Passed the old womans house where we staid night before last. She had sent a boy to us early this morning requesting us to pay him the 4 dollars due his mistress. We told him we did not know him and that he would go to his master for an order. He however followed us about a mile past his masters house when he returned back. Turned out at 3 to let our mules feed. Rain insued at 6 which turned to snow and what was still rode. We got ~~belated~~ hitched going over the Sand hills. We however continued sometimes in the road ~~and~~ & sometimes out until we reached a house where we were well entertained until morning Travelled 30 [miles].

Saturday 8th. Some rain this morning. Started at 1/2 past 8. Passed a small village called La Hoya[125] formed by a Fort but occupied at present by a miserable set of inhabitants. Obtained some ropes and passed on. Travelled 9 miles.[126] Night very cold with a stiff breeze.

Sunday 9th. Morning fine. Passed no inhabitants today. Put up at a ranch the last before the dry rout.[127]

Monday 10th. Morning fine. Some frost last night. Bot 2 sheep this morning to last us to the Pass. Travelled 20 miles. Encamped on the river bank.

Tuesday 11th. Cool last night. Started at sunrise. Travelled 15 miles encamped with a Spanish Caravan.

Wednesday 12th. Heavy dew last night. My mule was missing this morning. Rode back 1 1/2 miles [and] found him on the highlands.

---

[125]La Joya de Sevilleta, first mentioned by Juan de Onate in 1598, when he called the Piro Pueblo near here Nueva Sevilleta (New Seville). The pueblo site is on the bluff just a mile north of present-day La Joya. The present La Joya was founded in the 1790s by landless farmers from the northern part of the province. It had a fortified plaza by 1800, and when Zebulon Pike passed through in 1807, he was very impressed with the village, calling it "the neatest most regular village I have yet seen." Since La Joya was the last community before one reached El Paso del Norte, it was a collection point for caravans forming to enter the dangerous Jornada del Muerto. Jackson, *Following the Royal Road*, 57.

[126]The group camped near present-day San Acacia, New Mexico. The ruins of a Piro pueblo called Alamillo were noted by early Spanish travelers including Otermín, de Vargas, and Bishop Tamarón. However, the location of the Piro pueblo is not known today. Ibid., 58.

[127]The Jornada del Muerto.

Proceeded on 15 miles and encamped on the river. At this place we leave the river[128] and pack water. 80 miles before we strike the river again. Here we also cook to last us to the river.

Thursday 13th. Started this morning at daybrake. One of our mules failed but turn him lose and drive him.[129] Overtook the pack company at 3 Ock. Conclude to encamp for the night and send our mules to water 6 miles distant.[130] The men returned at 12 ock at night having left the tired mules near the river.

Friday 14th. Arrose by daylight this morning and assertain that 3 or 4 animals are missing and consequent to a thick fog did not find them until after sunrise. Reached the watering place a little after dark.

Saturday 15th. Started at 7. Reached the river at sunset much fatigued having walked a good part of the way. Found aplenty of fruit and spirits at the river.

Sunday 16th. Weather fine but cool nights and warm days. Did not touch this river again until night where we encamped in a grove and on the land granted to J. Heath[131] under certain provisions but now forfeited.

---

[128]Dr. Willard is at the paraje (camp site) called Fra Cristóbal, where the Camino Real leaves the river. Fra Cristóbal was one of the padres with Juan de Oñate in 1598.

[129]The *atajo* (the pack train of mules or burros) is part of a larger train that includes a *cavallada* or a herd of spare animals. Because the *mucho* (packed mule) could not carry the load anymore ("mule failed"), he was unpacked and turned loose into the *cavallada* to become a part of the larger drove until he recovered.

[130]Laguna del Muerto. Travelers had to utilize the water in the laguna if there was any or take the animals west down the arroyo to the Ojo del Muerto. This ojo, or spring, was found five miles west of the Camino Real. In 1863 Fort McRae was established near this dependable water source. Jackson, *Following the Royal Road*, 67.

[131]Dr. John G. Heath (1787–1847) was born in Pennsylvania. He was a wealthy lawyer who married Esther McDowell on July 4, 1814, in Saint Charles, Missouri. A later resident of Franklin, Missouri, he was an effective politician and businessman during the formative years when Missouri was promoting the settlement of the Boone's Lick country prior to achieving statehood. Heath was one of the thirty-five men of the Smithton Company who founded Smithton, which became Columbia, Missouri. As part of a well-connected, well-financed group of men, Heath knew of Moses Austin and his Texas colonization plan. Heath also knew William Becknell and other Santa Fe traders, which probably motivated Heath to apply to the Mexican government in 1822 for permission to found a colony at El Bracito, some thirty miles north of El Paso del Norte. The existence of a grove on Heath's land grant at the Camino Real paraje of

Monday 17. Cool and cloudy in the fore noon. Traveled 15 miles. Encamped near some sheep ranches.

Tuesday 18th. Left the waggons this morning and arrived at the Pass[132] at 1/2 after 12. Found the Americans in good spirits.

Wednesday 19. Conclude to leave with Mr. Campbell for Chauaua [Chihuahua] in the morning. Visited a gambling room in the evening. Staid until eleven. Mr. Ward lost about $150 but none myself. The game was monty.[133]

Thursday 18.[134] **[20]** Left El Paso[135] this morning at 8. Arrived at the Spring[136] at 5. Distance 35 miles. The distance from the pass to the next villiage[137] or settlement the Spaniards estimate to 40 odd leagues

---

El Bracito is also referred to by Samuel McClure, who wrote a letter to Col. M. M. Marmaduke from Cotton Grove and refers to Heath in his letter dated December 24, 1827. Unfortunately, when 150 colonists arrived from Franklin, Missouri, in 1824, Heath was informed that the grant had been repudiated. Most of the colonists returned to Missouri in 1825. By 1826 Heath, under penalty of death, was forced by the Mexican government to abandon all his personal property and leave the country. Heath returned to Missouri, bankrupt and financially ruined. It was alleged the venture cost him $75,000. Bowden, "John Heath Grant," New Mexico Office of the State Historian, http://dev.newmexicohistory.org/filedetails.php?fileID=24679 (accessed November 13, 2014); Sappington Papers, Missouri Historical Society.

[132]Again, El Paso del Norte.

[133]For a brief history of monte see Cady, *Loto*, 9.

[134]Starting on this date (Thursday, October 20, 1825), Dr. Willard's dates and days do not coincide. I have italicized them for the reader to reflect his confusion and resulting error while traveling El Camino Real.

[135]El Paso del Norte began as a religious community when the padres established a mission there in 1659. In 1680 it became a civilian town with the influx of the Pueblo Revolt refugees. The town thrived, growing to about five thousand inhabitants when Nicolás de LaFora visited in 1767. Zebulon Pike in 1807 reported the finely cultivated field of wheat and numerous vineyards producing "the finest wine ever drunk in the country." Today the city is known as Ciudad Juárez in honor of the republican president Don Benito Juárez (1806–72), who made El Paso del Norte his temporary capital in 1865 when the French drove the fleeing Juárez north. Jackson, *Following the Royal Road*, 89–91.

[136]The specific spring referred to is the Ojo de Samalayuca, a common and well-identified paraje on the Camino Real. It was subsequently mentioned by Adolph Wislizenus and others. The north face of the Sierra de Samalayuca contains a number of springs, although their flows have been greatly reduced by pumping for agriculture and industry.

[137]Carrizal or San Fernando las Amarillas del Carrizal was first sited in the 1700s as an agricultural and ranching settlement. The distances mentioned by Willard are about right. By the 1770s it was abandoned due to Indian attacks. A presidio was established there in 1773 with seventy soldiers. Josiah Gregg placed three to four hundred residents in Carrizal when he passed through in the 1830s. Today it is almost deserted. Jackson, *Following the Royal Road*, 108–109.

but the Americans 85 or 90 miles. Encamped at the Spring when Dr. Akins[138] overtook us.

Friday 19. [21] Rain last night. High winds. Having to pass through six or 8 miles [of] sandy roads. Conclude to tarry until the wind falls. Started late next day. Passed through the Sand hills[139] and encamped for the night. High wind which blows up rain.

Saturday 20. [22] Heavy rain last night and thru most of this day. Travelled 5 miles & encamped[140] where we succeeded in striking a fire.

Sunday 21. [23] Started again this morning at 8. Showers last night. Proceeded to the lake[141] and encamped.[142]

Monday 22. [24] Rain last night. Passed an uncomfortable night endeavoring to sleep in the waggons with three others.

Tuesday 23. [25] Started again at 7. Reached Carasal[143] abt 1/2 after 12: at this place the road forks. One heads to Chauauan the other to Sonora. My company take one and I the other.[144]

---

[138]William Aitken was one of the *albaceas* who witnessed the division of [trader] James Bairds' property at Ciudad Juárez, Chihuahua, on November 4, 1826. The other *albaceas* were John W. Rogers, Edward Beavers, Paul Anderson, and Samuel McClure. Dr. Aitken was a trader rather than a practicing doctor of medicine. Weber, *Taos Trappers*, 119.

[139]The Dunes of Samalayuca, immediately south of the Ojo de Samalayuca, are a major geographic feature on the Camino Real and cover an estimated two thousand square kilometers. Almada, *Diccionario*, 479. Caravans with heavy wagons generally avoided the dunes by taking a branch road along the south, or right, bank of the Río Bravo and the Arroyo de Cantareccio. Gregg also called them "Los Médanos, a stupendous ledge of sand-hills, across which the road passes for about six miles. As teams are never able to haul the loaded wagons over this region of loose sand, we engaged an atajo of mules at El Paso, upon which to convey our goods across. These Medanos consist of hugh hillocks and ridges of pure sand, in many places without a vestige of vegetation. Through the lowest gaps between the hills, the road winds its way." Josiah Gregg, *Commerce on the Prairies*, 274.

[140]This was probably Ojo de Lucero.

[141]Once known as the Laguna de San Miguel, today it is known as Laguna de los Patos [ducks]. The lake is 70 miles south of El Paso del Norte by the direct road and 96 miles by the one avoiding the sand dunes. Josiah Gregg, *Commerce on the Prairies*, 275.

[142]A common camping ground in this area was just to the south of the Sierra del Kilo or Sierra de la Candelaria on the edge of an arroyo that led from the sierra to the lake.

[143]The route from Carrizal to Sonora would go through La Ceja de Barrio, Galeana, Janos, and then over the mountains via either the San Luis or Pulpito passes.

[144]Ever fearful of attacks from bandits, many people formed convoys that traveled together and broke up as needed. Rondé, "Voyage," 144–61.

Wednesday 25. [26] Enjoyed a fair nights rest and the first since I left the Pass. Conclude to stay until tomorrow. Called on to visit a young woman, give her Physic. Her Brother agrees to carry my trunks to Chihuahua tomorrow. Attended a fangdango[145] last night but was not enamoured with the fair [ladies] of the City.[146] Their features are extremely course & their skin dark.[147] Left at 10.

Thurs. 26. [27] Morning fine. My company leave me this morning for Sonora.[148] Expected to have started early myself but my man has gone for his horses and dont return.

Friday 27. [28] Morning fine. Am still waiting for my man and his horses and with great impatients. Sr Hosen[149] called on me this morning and invited me to breakfast with him treating me with great attention. Called on me again to dine.

Saturday 30. [29] My man does not return yet with his horses. My friend persuades me to continue with him while I stay. Sends me a candle in the evening. Called on by a couple of young officers in the evening, who invited me home with them and to take a cup of chocklate.[150] Did so and spent the evening with them.

Sund. 31. [30] Attended church[151] this morning after which my friend called on me to breakefast with him. Did so [and] had a dish of pork the first I have met with in the country. Called on this morning by a young man from the Pass wishing me to accompany him to Chihuahua & offers me a horse. I consent. When I come to start my friend sent

---

[145]The arrival of travelers and/or their departure is reason enough to have a dance and throw a party.

[146]It is doubtful that in 1825 the population of Carrizal reached five hundred residents.

[147]This comment clearly reflects both the prejudices of the time and someone of Willard's background.

[148]The Camino Real also divides at this point with one branch following the course of the Río Carmen, and the other following a parallel but more easterly course. It seems as if Willard took the eastern branch.

[149]Josen.

[150]Chocolate, a luxury item then and now, has its origins in southern Mexico. A popular and medicinal drink for the last three millennia or more. The English word "chocolate" is derived from the Nahuatl word *xocolatl*, which means "bitter water."

[151]Many travelers attended church, not as a matter of principle but to follow the local norms.

me a basket of biscuit & cheese[152] for my journey. In this place Beard
Chambers & McKnight was imprisioned before the change of government.[153] Started at eleven and travelled until after dark probibly 25 or
30 miles and encamped in open prairie.[154] At 12 was awoken by the
running of horses.[155] I immediately arroused my man. When we salied
fourth to rescue our beasts found the horses but my mule was missing.
I mounted one horse in my drawers & my man the other and pursued
a mile or two but without success & returned. My man arrose again
at daybreak and went out and in half an hour returned with my mule.

1st of November. [October 31] Proceeded on our journey. Soon overtook a caravan with whom we conclude to keep company and camped
near a Spring[156] on the side of a mountains having travelled 30 miles.

Tues. Oct. Nov. 2d. [1] Started again this morning at 8. Travel 25 miles.
Encamped near Lake.[157] My mule threw his packs but did not brake
anything.

Wednesday 3? [2] Caught up this morning and proceed arrive to a little
town called Incinillas.[158] Encamped within a mile of it. Shower insued
at sunset but did not rain much.

Thurs. 4. [3] Morning cool. My mule missing this morning. Hunted
a mile or two distance arround but without success. Started without
her having obtained other animals from the company for my self and
baggage. The country here appears much more fertile than formerly.
Stopped at a ranch where we encamped for the night.[159]

---

[152]At the beginning of the twenty-first century, Carrizal and nearby Villa Ahumada are well
known for their asadero cheese.

[153]Chihuahua and New Mexico were still Spanish territory at this time.

[154]This could be close to either the Ojo de San Nicolas or Ojo de Santa Rosa.

[155]Horses were easily spooked by wild animals, lightning, and rustlers.

[156]This is Ojo del Gallego, a noted stop for caravans. It is situated to the east in the Sierra Gallego. Jackson, *Following the Royal Road*, 112.

[157]Laguna de Encinillas. See next note.

[158]Encinillas settlement was founded as a cattle ranch that provided fat and hides for the mines
of Santa Eulalia. It is on the edge of the ephemeral lake, Laguna de Encinillas.

[159]The location of the ranch is near where the Battle of Sacramento occurred in 1846.

Friday 5. [4] A part of the company leave us at this place. Proceeded within 2 leagues of Chihuahua[160] and encamped. Nights cool & days warm. Country looks dry and barren. Mountains mostly bare.

Sat. 6 Nov. [5] Arrived at Chihuahua much fatigued. This place is surrounded on 3 sides by low mountains[161] wholy destitute of timber and to an American traveler it is a matter of astonishment, on what this population subsist as there is scarcely a sign of aggraculture within 80 or 100 miles of the place.[162] Course hats are manufactured here, which is about all that can be said of manufacturers. The city is regularly laid out and tollerably well built though in the Spanish fashion.[163] Their buildings consist wholy of mud bricks & stones. They have some very good work of heavier stone particularly the Church which is a magnificent building wholly constituted of heavier stone and cost 300,000 dollars. It is built after the doric and corrinthian orders and with a great deal of ornamental carving. In it they have a large organ base drum and other instruments which accompanied with formal music constitutes the church melodies. Presented my letter of recommendation to Don Salvadore Porras[164] who treated me with a

---

[160]Today this spot would be lost under the urban sprawl of Chihuahua. It may have been at or near Nombre de Dios, the earliest Spanish settlement in the area (founded in 1697).

[161]To the east is the Sierra de Nombre de Dios, to the south Cerro Coronel (5,616 feet, named after Coronel Orozco y Molina who staked a claim on the edge of the hill in 1718) and Cerro Grande (6,371 feet).

[162]The areas propitious for farming are to the east of town after the Río Sacramento flows into the Río Chuviscar. The records of the Alhondiga (Municipal Granary) indicate that grains were frequently imported from as far away as Santa Rosalía (Santa Cruz, Tapacolmes) and the Papagochi valley.

[163]Chihuahua, founded in 1709 as Real de San Francisco de Cuellar, was made a *villa* (town) in 1718 with the new name San Felipe El Real de Chihuahua. Finally, in 1824, it was designated capital of the new Mexican state of Chihuahua with the simple name of Chihuahua. Sited at the confluence of the Ríos Chuviscar and Sacramento, this area was chosen to serve the nearby mines at Santa Eulalia. Corn and other agricultural products were brought in from agricultural zones in the foothills to the south and southwest. The downtown area has a fine cathedral, which was begun in 1727, consecrated in 1795, but not finished until 1826. During the period of 1825–47, the plaza was filled with commercial buildings used mainly for the camino traffic. Many ventures were foreign controlled: British, French, and American. Goods were brought here from Santa Fe, Mexico City, Veracruz, and Mazatlán and were shipped on to other towns and mining communities. Jackson, *Following the Royal Road*, 116.

[164]Salvador Porras was the ruler of Chihuahua during the struggle for independence led by Father Hidalgo. He was also a successful businessman as a trader and miner. His *(continued)*

great deal of politeness, gave me the charge of 5–6 rooms in which he caused my effects to be put.

Sunday 7. [6] Attended church this morning. Much amused with the Sacrisy and music. Found an old acquaintance O. Peck[165] and some other Americans which gives me much pleasure. My host has been trying ever since I came to get an interpreter to examine my papers but one is sick and the other is drunk.

Monday 8. [7] Called on to go before the Governor[166] this morning. Did so when he postponed examining them until Thursday at which time the Legislature[167] will be conviened.

Tuesday 9. [8] Weather somewhat cool but no fireplaces or wood in the country to speak of. Called on last evening, to visit a child having the malignant measels.[168] Gave it medicine but without much hopes of success.[169] Spend the most of my time with my American comps [companions].

Weds. 10th. [9] Hear my little patient has made its exit. Called on to give medicine to a man and his lady [and] did so.

Thurs. 11. [10] This day as near as I can learn my papers went before the Gov't Legislative body. The result I know not.

---

sympathies toward Hidalgo, who was shot in Chihuahua, resulted in his demotion and a fine. Porras served as a deputy in the Mexican Constituent Congress in 1822 and assisted three other deputies in drawing up a sixty-two-page memorial, which was completed in July 1822. The memorial described existing conditions and desirable changes for the western interior provinces of Mexico, including the need for provincial deputations for each western province. By December 1823 a provincial deputation had been authorized for Chihuahua. Nettie Lee Benson, *Provincial Deputation in Mexico*, 52–53, 59; Victor Orozco, *Estada de Chihuahua*, 68. It is also interesting to note that a son, José Salvador Serapio Porras Zubia, was born to Salvador Porras and his second wife, Gertrudis Zubia, on November 16, 1825, ten days after Dr. Willard's arrival in Chihuahua. FamilySearch.org (accessed September 7, 2011).

[165]Otis B. Peck, a carpenter and resident of Saint Charles, Missouri, when Dr. Willard lived there.
[166]Colonel José de Urquidi served from November 25, 1825, to February 27, 1826.
[167]This is the first session of the legislature of the state of Chihuahua.
[168]Willard may be referring to congenital rubella syndrome (CRS), a condition that occurs in an infant whose mother is infected with the virus that causes German measles.
[169]Nineteenth-century homeopathic medicine was even more hit-or-miss than today's allopathic medicine.

Friday 12. [11] Called on this morning to visit a couple of children one with measels the other debility [weakness]. Administered medicines.[170]

Satd. 13. [12] Visited my little patients this morning. Was presented with 4 dls [dollars]. Bought a pair of shoes gave $3. Spend most of the day with my Amn [American] friends. Mr. Peck is ornamenting my pistoles.[171] My culchions[172] nearly ready and other necessaries where I expect to keep house.

Sunday 14. [13] Attempted to pull a tooth for my landlord but was so cavious it broke off.[173] Visit a few patients this morning. Spend most of the day with my friends.

Mond 15. [14] Cool and cloudy. The *Serampion* or measles[174] are very previlent in this place, but few call for medical aid. Mr. Ferril[175] returns this evening.

Tuesday 16. [15] Obtain a *colchon* [mattress] and table today with some other necessaries, called on this eve to visit a young having the measles, a friend of my landlord. Yesterday accompanied Dr. Longar to examine a woman who died in child birth. Agreed that her death was caused by a malconformation of the pelvis.

Wednes. 17. [16] Called to visit one of my patients early this morning. Being highly exceeded with medicine his friends suposed him worse.[176] I however allayed their fears. Rain commenced last night and continued all day. Gave my friend Mr. Peck medicine to day who is

---

[170]It would be interesting to know what Willard prescribed since there is no known cure for measles except for bed rest and a calming topical.

[171]Assume Mr. Peck of Saint Charles was engraving his set of pistols.

[172]*Colchones* is the Spanish word for mattresses.

[173]The cavious tooth is pitted or rotten. Dentistry at this time was commonly left to barbers.

[174]*Sarampion* is the Spanish word for measles. While it is not known when the outbreak of measles began, it seems to have dissipated by the spring of 1826.

[175]Henry Ferril (1792–1854) was born in Kentucky and died in Miami, Saline County, Missouri. He was married to Martha Ferril and they had three children. William Becknell's company of 1822 (twenty-one men in all) included William Wolfskill, Henry Ferril, and Ewing Young. Wolfskill and Young remained in New Mexico. Barry, *Beginning of the West*, 106. Walter N. Gossler family tree and 1850 United States Federal Census, ancestrylibrary.com (accessed November 11, 2013).

[176]Overmedication has been with us for a long time.

much indisposed. Talked with Dn. Salvadore through an interpreter respecting my papers. He informs me that the Legislature are about to grant me and Dr. Longar license to practice. He said he will know the result tommorrow.

Thursday. 18. [17] Rained all last night and most of the day. Visit my patients today. No answer respecting my papers.

Friday 19. [18] Rained thru most of last night. My house leaks so bad that I am forced to leave it. Left it on Thursday [and] moved in with my American friends.

Satd. 20th. [19] Commenced bourding myself in company with Dr. Longar having a man & woman to cook.

Sunday 21. [20] Visited my patients this morning. Find them better. Recd. $10 this morning.

Monday 21.[177] Nothing of importance today. Save I was visited by a friend from St. Cruise John Anderson[178] by name. Bought of him a Buffalo robe.[179] Was visited by 3 gentlemen of the Legislature Petro Equisgoin,[180] Dn. Francisco Cordibe [Cordova], the other not known. They inform me they are about to do something with my papers and manifest a disposition to grant me licence.

Tuesday 22. Weather pleasant. Repair my trunks today & visit my patients.

Wednes 23. Nothing of importance today.

Thurs. 24. Dismissed all of my patients today. The weather has become fair and the measles less fatal.

Friday 25. Visited some ancient works above town where mineral was

---

[177]There are two entries. On Wednesday, December 21, 1825, Dr. Willard accurately synchronizes days and dates.

[178]Dr. Willard treated a John Andrews in Santa Cruz, New Mexico, on September 16, 1825. See n. 110.

[179]It is unclear if John Anderson is the person living in Santa Cruz and sold a buffalo robe, or if it is another person living in Santa Cruz, to whom Anderson sold a buffalo robe.

[180]Pedro José Irigoyen (1796–1864) was a member of the first Chihuahua state legislature. Almada, *Diccionario*, 284.

formerly smelted.[181] Examined an aqueduct of 50 arches[182] 15 or 20 ft high where water is brought to the town. There are 4 or 5 detached portions of similar magnitude said to be an ancient work but very well executed.

Sat 26. Got two or three new patients today. Nothing of importance.

Sund 27. Visited my patients as usual. Called to visit a young man son of an officer having the Sarampion.

Mond 28. Obtained two or three new patients today. The most of my patients are labouring under diarrha the relik of measles.

Tues. 29. Saw new patients today. Called on in the night to visit a child belonging to a Concubine of the Priest.

Wed 30. Weather cool but pleasant. No new patients today. The measles begin to abate. Nothing of importance today.

Thursday 1st December 1825. Snow falls all this day but melts nearly as fast as it falls.[183] Obtain one or two patients today. Have the care of ten or twelve complaints mostly consequent to measles.

Friday 2d. More pleasant. The snow melts fast. Obtain another patient today. Discharge 2 yesterday.

Sat. 3d Dec. 1825. Commenced bourding with John Finch[184] this day

---

[181]As Chihuahua was being founded a number of *haciendas de benificio*, or foundries, were built to make use of the water provided by the Río Chuviscar. From its beginnings, even before it was called Chihuahua, the local miners paid a self-imposed quota of five pesos to pay for the transport of ore from the mines to the southeast of Chihuahua to the foundries upstream. After 1738 these monies went directly to the coffers of the governors of New Viscaya. Ibid., 97.

[182]In 1751 the viceroy of New Spain ordered that these monies be recovered (stolen and then returned to the original owner) and, along with future revenue, be applied toward the construction of a system to provide drinking water to the growing town. The system grew in increments as the monies were diverted to support other projects. Forty years later, after a total investment in excess of $114,000, water was delivered to the fountain by way of the new stone aqueduct, still there today in the Plaza de Armas. Ibid., 11.

[183]Today, while not a yearly occurrence, snow is not unknown, and as in this case, it generally melts "as fast as it falls."

[184]Finch would seem to be Willard's general factotum. According to archival documents in Chihuahua, Juan Finch settled in Chihuahua in 1805. He was a tailor who also participated in the New Mexico trade. Finch married a local woman from Chihuahua in the parish church of San Felipe. Since Finch was bilingual, he had the potential to be a very useful person *(continued)*

at 12 1/2 dollars pr month. Appeard before the Governor today who grants me license to practice. Obtain 2 or 3 new patients today.

Sunday 4th. Called up early this morning to visit a patient. Obtain 3 others to day. Was called in by the priest who treated me very politely, advised him in his case it being the gravel. Mr. Griffith[185] arrives from the Pass.

Monday 5. Visit my patient. Discharge 3 of them. The rest are convelesent.

Tues. 6. Weather fine. The town was illuminated[186] last night consequent to the news having arrived by express that Saint John Alma[187] was relinquished by Old Spain.

Wednes. 7. On this day the feast commence. Much preperation in making by way of agrandisement. The city illuminated in the evening.

Thurs. 8. All Officers of Government appear in uniform today the evening beautifuly ehibiting illuminations and a variety of rockets.

Friday 9. This day the officer of State assemble in Congress Hall for the purpose of acknowledging the Constitution by oath. Was invited to witness the solemnity, did so. Illuminations & rockets[188] in the evening, much gaming at chuses in the public Square where men, women & children assemble.

Sat. 10. This day all of my American companions leave Chihuahua and

to have in one's employ. However, he was a drunk and prone to disappear for days at a time, causing Willard much inconvenience and even problems with the authorities. Martin, *Governance and Society*, 38–39.

[185]Robert Griffith (1791–1837) presented his factura on July 8, 1825, and was listed as an American foreigner from Columbia, Missouri. Weber, *Extranjeros*, 17.

[186]The principal source of light may have been something similar to *luminarias*.

[187]The fort of San Juan de Ulúa controls the entrance to Veracruz harbor. It was also known as Castle of San Juan de Ulúa, a large complex of fortresses, prisons, and one former palace on an island overlooking the seaport of Veracruz. It was the last redoubt of the Spanish army in Mexico and was surrendered by General Miguel Barragán in November 1825. "San Juan de Ulúa," http://en.wikipedia.org/wiki/San_Juan_de_Ul%C3%Baa (accessed September 7, 2011).

[188]Fireworks are a traditional component of religious celebrations in Mexico. Today fireworks are shot from each church and chapel to celebrate their patron saints' day, to honor the Virgin of Guadalupe, and to stimulate rain.

I left alone to spell out[189] the good and evil that awaits me. Witnessed this day a singular tradition. The dedication of the Guadalupe attended with most disgusting seremonies.[190] This may truly be called one of the dark corners of the earth.[191]

Sund. 11th. Sent for this morning to visit the principal Priest who is troubled with Gutta Serena.[192] Attended the ceremonies again today at the Temple—Called by the public Square which I found in a perfect uproar consisting of a mixed multitude engaged in gambling in a variety of ways. Here the rich and poor assemble in promiscus Crowds.[193]

Mond 12. The feasts still continue much firing of Canon & rockets today. Illumination at night. The people visit the temple again today to pay homage to the Guadalupe.[194]

Tues. 13. This is said to be the last day of the feasts. Mssrs. Beven[195] & Swene[196] arrive today. They put up with me while they stay.

Wed. 14. Nothing of importance today. Illuminates again tonight.

Thursday 15. Fel out with my landlord. Curse him and obtain a house of Capt. Martin who offers it me gratis.

Friday 16. Moove all of my effects today.

---

[189]"Spell out" in this context suggests the relief of one person by another in any work or duty. Webster, *Dictionary*, 2418.

[190]One may speculate that Dr. Willard was offended by the traditional dances performed by the *matachines*, which generally reflect a synchronistic vision of the conflicts between Christians and Muslims in Europe, and between Spaniards and Indians in the Americas.

[191]Willard clearly reflects the prevalent Protestant view that the Catholic Church has degraded itself by incorporating pagan elements.

[192]Idiopathic blindness, or blindness provoked by an unknown source.

[193]Willard probably would prefer to associate with what was then known as "a better class of people" rather than everybody.

[194]December 12 is the saint's day for our Lady of Guadalupe and would be the height of the celebrations and religious festivities.

[195]According to David J. Weber, Edward Beaven or Beaver(s) was issued a factura and guía #25 on August 22, 1825, in Santa Fe to sell his goods in Sonora. Weber, *Extranjeros*, 23–24. Edward Beavers was among the Americans who witnessed the division of James Baird's possessions in Ciudad Juárez after he had fallen sick and died in the Gila. Weber, *Taos Trappers*, 119.

[196]James Sweeney (1797–1842) was born in Lincoln, Kentucky. A year later, James G. Sweeney was issued guía #15 in his own name from the customhouse in Santa Fe sometime between the beginning of August and mid-September 1826. Weber, *Extranjeros*, 31.

Sat. 17. Nothing of importance today.

Sund 18. Attended church this morning. Was presented with a candle and in conformity to the Customs of the rest, marched around in form of procession occasionally kneeling to a representation of Christ—(the Eucharist) got out alive.

Mond 19. Nothing of importance today.

Tues. 20. Visited the Temple with Messers Bevers & Sweeney. Also the ancient aquiducts said to have been commenced at an early day by the Jesuits.[197]

Wednes. 21. Cloudy this morning. Nothing of importance.

Thursday 22. My comrades leave me this morning for Durango.[198] Send a letter by them to P. Wetmore.[199] The Priest whose eyes I have treated is so much better that he has left town for St. Cruise. Paid me 24 dollars & expressed much satisfaction.

Friday 23. Lost a patient last night who sunk under debility before I was called. Have been called to 3 new patients today, two yesterday.

Satday 24th. Hear from my friends at N. Mexico by a Spaniard directly from there. All of my patients convelesent save one P. Woman laboring under Pneumonia with obstination degeneration.[200]

---

[197] The Jesuits built their own college and chapel that later served as the military hospital, foundry, mint, and museum, but there is no evidence that they were involved with the construction of the aqueduct and water system.

[198] Durango, first named Guadiana, was sited in 1563 by Francisco de Ibarra. Ibarra was a nephew of Diego de Ibarra, one of the four founders of Zacatecas. Diego de Ibarra's silver mining fortune financed his nephew Francisco's explorations of the Guadiana valley. Nicolás de LaFora, a soldier and explorer who visited Durango in 1766, said there were thirteen hundred families of españoles, mulatos, and mestizos and one quarter or section of Durango with ninety-five families of Indians. When Josiah Gregg visited Durango in 1835, he called it one of the handsomest cities in the north, with two or three attractive plazas and some twenty thousand residents. Jackson, *Following the Royal Road*, 142.

[199] On August 22, 1827, Alphonso Wetmore, a well-known Santa Fe trader, received guías #7 and #10, respectively, to take merchandise to Chihuahua along with Henrique Connully [Henry Connelly] and Santiago Glenn [James Erwin Glenn]. Weber, *Extranjeros*, 33. P. Wetmore is identified as living in San Luis Potosí in Willard's diary entry from July 14, 1826.

[200] Possibly an obstinate diarrhea or a kidney or spleen degeneration. Senator, Litten, and Herrick, *Diseases*, 562.

Sund 25. My pneumonia patient is better today. Her friends fearing her disolution was near, Confessed & administered to her the Sacrament.

Mond 26. My patients all convelescent. A procession was formed this afternoon headed by music and a small image resembling the Virgin Mary bore on the shoulders of four men.[201] She was richly decorated, with candles in glass lanthons lighted around her. She was crowned with gold and bespangled with jewels, before this image of wax they bow in adoration.

Tues 27. Cloudy and cool. Rained in the evening. Wrote to my friend Houck[202] today.

Wedns 28. Wrote to Mr. Anderson[203] at St. Fee by Mr. Cordiva— nearly all of my patients are off my hands.

Thurs. 29. Samething indisposed today having caught a bad cold. Principal Priest[204] paid me $44 today.

Dec. 30. John Anderson from New Mexico paid me a visit to day. Send by him a letter to St. Fee.

Sat. 31. Samething indisposed from a bad cold. This day the Govt. Body sent me my licence to practice, requiring me at the same time to visit the poor gratis & give advice but not medicine.[205]

---

[201]While it is a common act of veneration to take statues from churches and parade them through the streets and then place them in a private home or a public place to be worshipped, it is not clear why the day after Christmas would have been chosen.

[202]Solomon Houck (1802–72) was born in Virginia. He moved to Kentucky and eventually on to Boonville, Missouri. He was a trader on the Santa Fe Trail and lived in Mexico for a time. On October 14, 1826, guía #21 was issued to Houck and Inby. Weber, *Extranjeros*, 31. Solomon Houck was with "The company of traders (size unknown) which left Fort Osage in August (1826) and reached Santa Fe in November included James Collins (at a later date Indian affairs superintendent in New Mexico), Elisha Stanley, Solomon Houck, Edwin M. Ryland, James Fielding, Thomas Talbott, and William Wolfskill. All these men remained in Mexico for nearly a year." Barry, *Beginning of the West*, 135. Solomon Houck was identified as a prominent Santa Fe merchant who helped finance Ewing Young's beaver hunts in 1828. Weber, *Taos Trappers*, 141.

[203]William (Bill) Anderson lived in Santa Fe. Dr. Willard also met his brother Colonel Paul Anderson, who was part owner of the steamboat *Uncle Sam* in New Orleans. See Willard's autobiography, page 242.

[204]It is not clear if Principal Priest refers to the same person that is subsequently identified as P. Padre, Cura, or Padre Anchondo.

[205]Unfortunately, the Chihuahua State Archives burned down more than fifty years ago. All documents, such as those relating to Willard's and Longar's applications for medical licenses, were destroyed.

Sund 1st Jan 1826. This is a day of feasting and rejoicing. A scrumptious dinner was prepared for the nobility. Had the honor of an invitation, accepted, was treated with much politeness. Fangdango in the evening but to unwell to attend.

Monday 2d. My interpreter gits drunk and bothers me. A few new patients.

Tues. 3. Nothing of importance today.

Weds 4. Weather more pleasant.

Thurs. 5th. Messers Beavers & Sweeney return from the Parral[206] today.

Friday 6. Write to Dr. Millington[207] by Messrs Beavers & Sweeney. My patients all better.

Sat 7. My companions[208] leave this afternoon for the Pass not being able to practice below for the want of license. Purchase all of their medicines for forty dollars.[209]

Sund 8. Regulate[210] my medicines to and visit my patients as usual.

---

[206]Parral, also known as San José de Parral and Hidalgo de Parral, is a major mining center in the southern part of the state. In the eighteenth century it was the de facto capital of Nueva Vizcaya due to the silver mines in the area. "Pedro Rivera who visited Parral on an inspection tour of frontier defenses in 1726, commented that it had 'considerable mining in times past' and noted that at that time, it was the residence of the governor and *capitán general* of Nueva Vizcaya." Jackson, *Following the Royal Road*, 133.

[207]Jeremiah and Seth Millington were brothers from New York, both physicians. They were two of the first doctors to settle in Saint Charles. Together they owned fifty acres of castor beans and produced the first commercial castor oil, which they shipped all over the world. They supplied the medicine for the Lewis and Clark expedition in 1804. Jeremiah also served as the Saint Charles postmaster when Saint Charles was the state capital of Missouri. Stewart and Knox, *Earthquake America Forgot*, 126. An advertisement in the *Missourian* newspaper from Saint Charles dated April 25, 1821, states: "Doctor Millington, Continues the practice of *Medicine, Surgery, and Midwifery*, in the town of St. Charles, and its vicinity. Those who may call will find him at his brick house, second door below the Kentucky Hotel. June 24th, 1820." The same issue also lists Seth Millington as a trustee of the Saint Charles Academy, which was established by an act of the General Assembly of the state of Missouri passed November 16, 1820.

[208]Willard's companions were Beavers and Sweeney leaving for El Paso del Norte.

[209]Exchange of merchandise, medicines, and later negatives was a common practice between traders, doctors, and photographers.

[210]Willard probably checked the strength, color, and viscosity of his homemade remedies.

Mond 9. Messrs Storrs Williams[211] and Parrish[212] arrive. Visit the Customs house where their goods were examined.

Tues 10. Visited the Temple with my companions who were much pleased with the splendor and tast of workmanship.

Wed 11. Visited my patients this forenoon, afternoon. Paid several visits with my friend Stoors.

Thurs. 12. Mr. Stephens[213] arrives today. Dr. Akins will be here in the morning.

Frid 13. This day a complaint was entered to me against my comrades for not having knelt and pulled of their hats while their Host[214] was passing by. I patched the offence by saying I was fully sensible they were unacquainted with the intention of the procession.

Sat. 14. We again visited the Temple in order to take a description of its exceeding beauty. But from the complications of the architecture considered ourselves incompetent.[215]

Sund 15. Had several professional calls today. Attended church with the rest of my companions. We were all presented with a candle where we were required according to the custom of the rest to form

---

[211]Willard does not include sufficient information to establish which Williams he is talking about. It could be Ezekiel, Isaac, Joseph, William, or even somebody else who has not been identified in the literature. Weber, *Taos Trappers*, 262.

[212]John E. Parrish was issued guía #26 in 1825 to take merchandise to Sonora and Chihuahua. Weber, *Extranjeros*, 24. John G. Parrish was one of the witnesses to the division of James Baird's material possessions in Ciudad Juárez during the first week of November 1826. Weber, *Taos Trappers*, 119.

[213]A man named Stevens partnered with Baird and Chambers in building the distillery at Taos. In the spring of 1831 Jefferson Blackwell and John Gantt led a party up the Platte River; "K. Stephens, who had once been to Santa Fe," was one of their subalterns. Weber, *Taos Trappers*, 72.

[214]On the whole the foreigners would have been Protestants; they were thus unaware of and were uninterested in Catholic sensibilities. This comment suggests that Willard interacted with some of the more conservative elements of the local society and was seen as, or wished to play the part of, a cultural mediator. When he first arrived in Chihuahua, Willard was openly antagonistic to the Catholic rituals and ceremonies, but as he became more familiar with the rituals and developed friendships with the people and priests, his aversion diminished.

[215]Philippe Rondé is the first person known to have drawn the façade of the church in 1849. Rondé, "Voyage," 137.

a procession and march around the church occasionally falling down to the priest who bore in his hand a representation of the sun made of gold.[216]

Monday 16. Recd an invitation to visit the governor in Company with the rest of the Americans.[217] His object appeared to be no more than to see Mr. Storrs the Consul, as he requested his commission. Dr. Akins is packing up for Sonora.

Tues 17. Another complaint was alledged against one of my fellow Americans for not having pulled his hat at the sound of the bell.

18. Called on today to visit the Legislation Hall and then to give in our names and occupations, also our places of residence and business in this country.[218] The Governor had the commission of our Consul interpreted and translated into Spanish. Another remarkable circumstance took place our companion Dr. Akins having sent out for a bottle of whisk[219] and invited his companions to drink with him.

Thurs 19. Nothing of importance today.

20. Dr. Akins leaves today for Sonora, having sold but few goods in this place. Gave my interpreter who had been drinking several days a few portions of Tart Emt[220] in his draws.

21. Consul Storrs has been indisposed several days which proved to be the measles.[221]

---

[216]This would be the monstrance (*custodia* or *ostensorio* in Spanish) used to hold the host, the wafer representing the body of Christ in a Mass.

[217]It would seem as if the governor was taking the opportunity to inform the American consul and most foreigners of the need to register for the annual census of foreigners. By the 1840s the process had become quite formal, and all foreigners were expected to carry a *carta de seguridad* to demonstrate the legitimacy of their presence in Mexico.

[218]The actual registration for the census.

[219]It is not clear if Willard was surprised that Dr. Aitken sent for a bottle of whiskey, found one, or shared it. However, since Dr. Aitken was about to leave for Sonora, it does not seem surprising that a celebration was in order.

[220]Willard gave Mr. Finch a dose of tartar emetic or antimonium tartaricum (antimony potassium tartrate), an emetic to induce vomiting and clean out Mr. Finch's system. Rothstein, *American Physicians*, 52.

[221]This was the first case of the measles in more than a month, according to Dr. Willard.

22d. Was presented with a crats [cravat] cloth today by my friend Dn. Salvadore.

23. Discharged 4 of my patients which have had a course of nervous fever. Friend Storrs much better.

24. Nothing of importance today.

Wed 25. Do Do Do Do Do.[222]

Thurs 26. Friend Storrs has recovered from the measles[223] and able to walk out.

Frid 27. Nothing of importance.

Sat 28. Visit my patients as usual. Much wind from S.W.

Sund 29. Messers Storrs & Parrish more unwell today than usual.

Mond 30. Killed two ravens with the pistols. Visited my patients as usual.

Tues 31. Nothing of importance.

Wednes 1st Feb. Finch in another Spree.

Thus 2d. Take Finch to my room & set him to work to keep him sober.

Frid 3. Snow and rain today.[224]

Sat 4. The storm still continues but melts nearly as fast as it comes.

Sund 5. Snow 3 or 4 inches deep this morning. Weather continues foul.

Mon 6. Went before the Alcalde today for giving my interpreter a salutary & merited chastisement.[225] Trial adjourned to tomorrow morning.

Tues. 7. Appeared before the Alcalde this morning but my interpreter ordered the trial to be discontinued. Weather fine today.

---

[222]"Ditto," abbreviated "do."

[223]A quick recovery. The normal course of measles seems to be anywhere from one to three weeks.

[224]The second snowstorm produced more snow, lasted longer, and was colder than the previous storm on December 1.

[225]Evidently Willard was unable to control his temper. Finch's general drunkenness annoyed and frustrated Willard, who seems to have given Finch a cuffing.

Wed 8. Rode out this evening and on returning home was thrown from my horse who made his escape to the mountains. Gave a boy a dollar to return him.

Thus. 9. Weather cool. Visited Senr. Severena[226] with Col. Storrs today, who treated us very politely and presented me with 50 dollars as a compensation for my services. Gave her back 15. Not expecting more than 20.

Frid 10. The Lawyer called on me today his wife being a little indisposed. Requested my bill which was two ds. He gave me six.

Sat 11. Again appeared before the Alcalde with my interpreter who told his story to suit his case whereupon the court fined me $20.

Sund 12. My countrymens horses which have been lost 2 weeks are brot in. This is the day of Guadalupe it being the 12 Dec.[227]

Mond 13. Rode out today and on my return my horse jumped and threw me and made his escape. A soldier volunteered and herded him 9 miles and brought him back.

Tues 14. Rode out again today my horse more gentle.

Wednes 15. My companions are preparing to start for New Mexico. Write by them to my Father, two Sisters, My Preceptor, Mr. Postal,[228] and Solomon Houck. Was visited in the evening by the family of Sr. Escudero[229] now in the U. States.

Thus 16. This day my countrymen take their departure having sold to the amt of 4 or 5 hundred dls.

---

[226]Doña Severena is identified as Dña Sae, Seva, Soverena, and Serverena.

[227]Although the saint day for the Virgin of Guadalupe is the 12th of December, religious zealots celebrate the Virgin of Guadalupe on the twelfth of every month to a lesser degree.

[228]William Postell was one of the men Willard worked with as a carpenter in New York. He traveled with Dr. Willard to Saint Charles in 1817. Willard visited Mr. Postell and his family in June 1828 after he returned to the United States. He then went on to Palmyra and Dorset, New York, to visit his family, whom he hadn't seen in more than ten years.

[229]Escudero is Manuel Simón de Escudero, according to an email communication from David Weber on November 30, 2009.

Frid 17. Feel somewhat lonely being confined to the Spanish language and unable to speak it.

Sat 18. Spend most of the day in reading. Have had few patients.

Sund 19. Attended church this morning, high wind from south.

Mond. 20. Feel a little indisposed today. As near as I can learn Spain had sent a force of 4,000 men to the Havana for its protection.

Tues 21. Recommence boarding with John Finch. Visit my patients as usual.

Wednes. 22. My interpreter in his ways again. Went a Crowing with my pistols.

Ths. 23rd February 1826. Have many calls from the Poor who solicit me in the name of my namesake Saint, to tell them of some remedy for their infirmaties.

Frid 24. My interpreter still in his frolic made many visits today.

Sat 25. Weather beautiful indeed. Took a letter out of the Office directed to Otis Peck. Expecting it was from P. Wetmore but found it was from Dn. Russell Saltillo.[230] Several female visitors today.

Sund 26. Several new patients of mostly cronic complaints. Have two or three cases of dropsy.

Mond 27. The same routine of visiting and having the doleful tales of infirmaty. Took a game of cards with Messrs. G.

Tues 29. Gave my interpreter an emetic last night in order to sober him. Is rational today. Have several old women under pills and bitters. Was advised by a lady from St. Heronamo[231] upon the propriety of her fasting during lent she being in delicate health thought a deliterious

---

[230]Unknown person.

[231]San Heronimo or Jeronimo is now known as Juan Aldama, the county seat of the Municipio de Aldama, Chihuahua. It lies about thirty-five kilometers to the northeast on the road to Ojinaga, which is across the border from Presidio, Texas.

and confessed to the Priest the omission of that duty. Whereupon he required her to ask my opinion in the case which should decide whether she was committing an offence pardonable or unpardonable. Decided that she should eat!

Wed. 1st March. Spent the day in getting instruments made. At night called to three or four new patients, one of which had sent for the Priest befor me though he arrived a little after. When I was requested to leave the room until she the patient should confess. I replied that I should go to my room if I went out, and if they prefered the priest to the Doctor to confess, if not to take the medicine then, or I should not give it at all. She thereupon took it. I then told the priest if they was all agreed they might confess and left there.

Thurs 2d. Was called up last night at 12 Ock the Alcalde having sent for me to visit a man whom a woman had stabed with a knife. When found him a large portion of the omentum[232] had protruded at the orifice and the patient continually retching as if to void stomach and all its contents. I succeeded in reducing the viscus by enlarging the orifice where I secured it by sutures and compress. Visited him this morning. Find him something easier though much exercised with pain in the region of the abdomen. Several new patients today. Took a game of cards with Miss. G_____.

Frid 3. Discharged four patients to day. My wounded man still alive & to appearance some better. Got a trocar[233] and other instruments made today, in order to perform Paracentesis.[234]

---

[232]"Omentum is a sheet of fat that is covered by the peritoneum. The greater omentum is attached to the bottom edge of the stomach, and hangs down in front of the intestines. Its other edge is attached to the transverse colon. The lesser omentum is attached to the top edge of the stomach, and extends to the undersurface of the liver." MedicineNet.com, http://www.medterms.com/script/main/art.asp?articlekey=4632 (accessed November 11, 2009).

[233]A trocar is a sharply pointed shaft, usually with a three-sided point. A trocar may be used within a cannula, a hollow tube, designed to be inserted into a vein, artery, bone marrow, or body cavity. The word "trocar" is derived from the French "trois" (three) + "carre" (side). MedicineNet.com, http://medterms.com/script/main/art.asp?articlekey=20090 (accessed October 20, 2009).

[234]"The operation of tapping facilitates the evacuation of the collected fluid in ascites [abdominal dropsy], ovarial dropsy, &c." Dunglison, *Medical Lexicon*, 551.

Sat 4. Peach trees are in blossom and leaves fill out to a considerable size. Have many calls for charity from the Poor. Represented to one of the principal alcaldes the impropriety of giving the Spanish Dr. a Sallery for doing nothing and at the same time requesting me to advise the poor for nothing!

Sund 5. Weather somewhat cooler today. Paid Miss. A. a visit today who made me many threats for having absented myself so long.

Mond 6. My wounded man still seems to get better. Interpreter in another frolick. Day cloudy with some rain at night.

Tues 7. Called on to visit a patient of Dr. Lopez. Refused to give medicine without his consent and left him.

Wed 8. Called on last night to visit several at St. Michael & St. Lorenzo[235] 50 miles distant. Started at 8. Arrived at 1/2 past 7. Much fatigued. Found my patients very sick, staid with them 2 days. Left them on the 3d for St. Magil with an express from the Priest at that place. He having a touch of the apoplexy.[236] Staid with him over night, was treated exceedingly kind.

Sund 12. Left St. Magil at 8. Arrived at Chihua_ a little after 4. Had 2 or 3 calls to the sick before I got into my room much fatigued.

Mond 13. Had several professional calls today. My patients appear to be glad at my return. Some having cried in my absence.

14. March. Two or three new patients today. Cura Nava[237] commenced a course of medicine for venerial this eve.

15. Attend mostly to my books having but few patients.

16. My interpreter is missing. His family knows nothing of him.

---

[235]There is a San Miguel de los Anacondas and a San Lorenzo in close proximity to Santa Isabel in the Municipio de General Trías. The distances are a little more than fifty miles, but that would be a fair approximation.

[236]Apoplexy or apoplexia is uncontrolled bleeding leading to excessive strokes. See Dary, *Frontier Medicine*, 42.

[237]Nava was a common surname in Chihuahua. Fray Angelico Chávez refers to two types of Catholic curas: *cura propio* and *cura encargado*. See n. 69. Chávez, *But Time and Chance*, 25–26.

Thunder shower this evening. Recd a letter from Dr. Akin for medicines.

17. Priest Anchondo[238] sent me his compliments this morning before I was up. Informing me that he had arrived, and solicited my visits— Was visited by several Women in the evening.

Sat. 18. Was called up last night at 12. My interpreter has taken his departure to the South in a clandestine manner.

Sund 19. Nothing of importance.

Mond 20. Had a call this morning before I got up to visit a woman at St. Cruise,[239] but some of my patients were opposed to it, and I declined.

Tues. 21st. Patients from the country with Cronic complaints of long Standing.

Wed. 22. High wind which overwhelmed the town in dust. This is the week dedicated to the Saints &c.[240]

Thus. 23. This is a great day[241] among the Christians and is commemorated as the anniversary of the death of *Christ*. Had a sermon this evening delivered by my good friend Anchondo. A procession insued. Was invited to dine with Dn. Salvadore Porras. Accepted. Called to dress a wound one woman received by a knife in the hands of another female.

Frid 24. Another sermon,[242] today they crucify their Lord and entomb him. A procession was afterwards formed, in which the sepulcre[243] containing the body was bore on shoulders, also two angels on the right

---

[238]Rafael Anchondo (1786–1837) was born in Satevó, Mexico. He studied for the priesthood in Durango, where he took his vows. At one stage he was the priest in both Cusihuiráchi and Allende. He was elected *diputado* in 1832 and died in 1837. Luis Urias Hermosillo, personal communication, October 2009.

[239]Probably Santa Cruz de Tapacolmes.

[240]This is the first day of Holy Week.

[241]Maundy Thursday is the fifth day of Holy Week and the celebration of the Last Supper. Dr. Willard seems to have missed the reason Don Porras invited him to supper.

[242]Good Friday.

[243]A sepulcher is a casket or coffin.

and left[244] and this surrounded by a rabble in wampom[245] uniform representing the Faricus.[246] In the rear followed by the virgin Mary and St. John the Evangelist. Many bearing crosses of an enormous weight. A confused rabble.[247]

Sat. 25 March. This is the resurrection day and close of the feast.[248] The enormous mockery and superstition has subsided a little.[249]

Sund 26. Visited 12 or 15 patients today besides several who visited me.[250] Have but little time to read. My patients all amending.

Mond 27. Several calls before out of bed this morning. Several new patients and a vareity of diseases Gonorrhea, hives, fever, dropsy, Dispepsia, wounds, fistula,[251] Apoplexia, Palpitations, diseases of infants, and old age.

Tues. 28. Bastantas infirmous.[252]

Wed. 29. Several new cases today. Was called to visit a woman under colic[253] when I found Dr. Lopes who seamed to decline giving prescription and left. I accordingly administered relief.

---

[244]Pairs of "small angels on the left and right" held the ends of a long cord (*la soga*) around Jesus's neck. Alternately, two criminals, later named Gestas and Dismas, one of them blaspheming Jesus and the other defending him, appeared in the Gospel of Luke 23:35–42. Father Thomas J. Steele S.J. and Felipe R. Mirabel, correspondence to author, October 2009.

[245]Wampon or wampum usually refers to shells and their use as money, or in rare occasions as adornments. In this specific case, Dr. Willard would seem to be referring to mummers or dancers known as *concheros* (rough translation: people of shells) that traditionally decorate their costumes with shells and use large shell bracelets and anklets. Today, *concheros* tend to hold indigenous rather than Christian beliefs.

[246]Pharisees.

[247]For those that know the thread, there is order in chaos.

[248]Dr. Willard seems to be confused, or the local residents may be working on a different religious calendar. While Holy Saturday is the last day of Holy Week and as such the body of Christ lies in his tomb, it is on the third day, Easter or Holy Sunday, that he rises again.

[249]Dr. Willard reveals his anti-papist perspective.

[250]This suggests that a "normal" roster of patients would be about twenty.

[251]A fistula is an abnormal connection between an organ, vessel, or intestine or another structure. Fistulas are usually the result of injury or surgery and can also result from infection or inflammation.

[252]Pidgin Spanish for "many ill people."

[253]Colic in adults is defined as paroxysmal pain in the abdomen or bowels.

Thur. 30. Nothing of importance Save I lost a patient under advanced stage of pleurisy, having been called to late to save her.

Friday 31st. Nothing of importance.

Satur. 1st April 1826. Several new cases today and of a difficult and doubtful nature.

Sund 2d. Arroused every morning by patients. Some send their servants to know if they can attend church, others if they are well enough to leave their bed &c. Recd two boxes of goods consigned to me from Mr. Floid. Sundry presents from the old woman.

Mond. 3d. Nothing of importance. The Lieutenant called on me for medical aid he not having confidence in the Hospital Dr.[254]

Tues 4th. Nothing of importance.

Wed 5. Messrs Douglas[255] and West[256] arrive today with goods.

Thus. 6. Visited the temple this eve and my patients as usual.

Frid 7. Dismissed several patients. Am frequently solicited to be baptised and marry in this country, particularly by the old women who lament that I not a Christian.

Sat 8 Apr. Much wind and dust all day.

Sund 9. Attended church in the morning. Visited my patients in the evening.

Mond. 10. Cool and Pleasant.

---

[254]The military hospital was probably housed in the old Jesuit Convent. Father Miguel Hidalgo and the other revolutionaries were held prisoner in the old Jesuit Convent before they were shot.

[255]James [Burnsides] Douglas[s] (1785–1854) was born in Madison, Kentucky, and died in Johnson, Missouri. He was an American merchant and resident of Parral, Chihuahua, as noted in the census of 1831. Willard's reference to his death in Santa Fe is incorrect.

[256]In Governor Narbona's February 1, 1826, Report on Foreigners, Gorge [George] Weste's occupation is listed as cabinet maker. In the book of guías West was granted a guía in 1826. In the Treasury Reports/Santa Fe/1826–1827 listed among the outgoing funds during September 1826 is a payment to Santiago Douglass and Jorge Westt, which represents the return of a deposit paid at Chihuahua. Weber, *Extranjeros*, 27, 31.

Tues. 11. El Pad[re] Anchondo arrives to day on his way to the hot spring[257] where I agreed to accompany him but at present out of my power.

Wed 12. Sundry patients under cronic diseases.

Thus. 13. Discharge my cook today and commence keeping house in company with my two companions.

Frid. 14. Commence giving a Lady med. for Secondary Leus.[258]

Sat 15. Lost an aged patient today, the rest convelesent. Recd a letter from P. Wetmore at St. Louis Potosi.

Sund 16. Attended church this morning. Returned home much fatigued from kneeling.

17. Had a controversy with the relations of a diceased whom I have doctored better than 3 months. She having died ~~almost~~ insolvent. They appropriately rising $50 for her burial and pay me nothing for my services whereupon I remonstrate and claim my services.

Tues 18. Something indisposed today from bad cold.

Wed 19. Have generaly 18 or 20 patients to prescribe for every day from ten to fifteen of which are regular patients.

Thus. 20. Nothing of importance.

Frid. 21. A small shower with some thunder in the evening.

Sat 22. Nothing of importance.

Sund 23. The Spaniards spend the Sabbath in gaming in a variety of ways though principaly in cock fighting.[259] A hundred dollars was bet on one game today.

---

[257]San Diego de Alcalá hot springs are located to the southeast of Chihuahua and about 15 km due east of Bacimba. On May 7, 1826, when he took his second trip to the springs, Dr. Willard identified the distance as thirty-five miles.

[258]Syphilis.

[259]Cockfighting is still a popular sport in Mexico. By 1850 there was a cockfighting pit in Plaza Merino, behind what was the parish church.

Mond 24. Expect to start in the morning for the Springs.[260] Deposited $525 with Dn. Bissenta Bissenta [Vicente de Vicente] for safe keeping.

Tues 25. Started this morning with a coach & seven in company. Mr. Douglass & Col. Arsas[261] wife and sister for the Springs. Dined at Dolores. Arrived at San Diego at Sun Set where we found El Padry Anchondo & family.

Wed. 26. Visited the Springs this morning. These Springs are of the temperature of 150 or two hund. F.F. impregnated with iron sulpher. Sodas &c.

Thus. 27. Return to Chihuahua. Arrive at 3 Ock. Visit my patients.

Frid 28. Several patients groaning under moderate salivations for Lues veneria.

Sat. 29. Nothing of importance.

Sund. 30. High wind all day and night. Ex. Padery returns today.[262]

Mond. 1st May. Myself & countrymen recd. an invitation to dine, accepted. Today they commemorate the birth of St. Philip. High winds. Recd. a letter from Joshua Griffiths at the Pass. Put a letter in the office for P. Wetmore.

Tues 2d. Feel quite indisposed from bad cold.

---

[260]San Diego de Alcalá Springs.

[261]In Willard's diary he is subsequently referred to as Colonel Azar on Sunday, May 7, 1826. It would seem Colonel Arsas or Azar is Lt. Col. José Antonio Arce, who after a distinguished military career became the second governor of Chihuahua. Col. Arce spent most of his career in the military posts in and around Chihuahua and New Mexico. He was named the senior military officer in Chihuahua in 1823 and was known to be living there as of the middle of 1825. He was appointed vice governor by the state legislature and, as of September 26, 1825, took over the role of governor, which he ceded to Coronel Urquidi on November 26, 1825, when he assumed the presidency of the Council of State. He continued to be active in political affairs with his election as vice governor in 1826. Shortly thereafter, due to the absence of the elected governor, Simón Elías González, Arce resumed the post of governor from February 27 to September 25, 1826, when González returned to Chihuahua. Barely a month later, González resigned and José Antonio Arce again took over the governorship. For more details see Almada, *Diccionario*, 43–44.

[262]This could be a reference to Padre Anchondo. "Ex" would seem to be an abbreviation for *su excelencia*, a title given to bishops. Chihuahua did not become a diocese until the propagation of *La bula Illud in primis*, on the June 23, 1891, by Pope Leo XIII. Vázquez, *Fundación de la Diócesis*, 3.

Wed 3. Nothing of importance. Drew from Dn. Besenta $31. Purchas 26 fine hats of Mr. Douglas for $156.[263]

May 4. Mssrs. Douglas and West leave for the Pass having sold to the amt of $1,800.

Frid 5. Am informed that I shall probably be appointed to direct the Hospital as a complaint has been instituted against the present Physician for neglect of duty and a supposed incompetency to manage it.

Sat 6. But few patients at present.

Sund 7. Receive an invitation to ride to the Springs[264] today. Accept in company with Col. Arza family he having prepared a coach and seven for our conveyance. Started at 8. Arrived at 5. Distance 35 miles.

Mond. 8. All visited the Springs and baths. Afternoon recreate ourselves with cards and walking.

Tues 9. Returned to Chiha. Arrived at 6 A.M. visit my patients. Recd 8 or 10 female visits in the evening.

Wed. 10. Several new patients under venerial. Receive many visits morning and evening. Compliments from the Priest at St. Pablio today.

Thus. 11. May. Was warmly solicited to be Baptized a Roman Catholic by one of the first families of the place. Put them off by urging the necessity of understanding their language & Church discipline. Was presented with a gold piece Handkerchief &c by a Lady.[265]

Frid. 12. Was informed last evening that the Ayuntemento[266] was a little dissatisfied considering that I'm not charitable to the poor. When

---

[263]Each hat cost six dollars, and since Douglas and West left Chihuahua the next day, one can imagine that Dr. Willard was looking for a "good buy" so that he too could turn a penny.

[264]San Diego de Alcalá hot springs.

[265]This suggests that Dr. Willard has received a certain level of social acceptance as a person. In order to really integrate himself into Chihuahuan society (in other words, to prove his moral worth and commit himself to local values), he would be expected to convert to Catholicism. By the end of the nineteenth century a number of mainstream leading families (e.g., Luis Terrazas) incorporated foreign males (e.g., Russek and Creel) who appeared as traders or military men (e.g., Cuilty).

[266]The ayuntamiento is the municipal corporation generally composed of the alcalde and the consejales or regiadores (council).

I assured them that I bestowed more charity than any other man in the place according to my means. And if they were not pleased with my conduct they might find another Phisician, for I asked them no favors. Arreigned a Sergent before the Major for failure in payment and false promises. He agrees to detain his wages to the Aunt.[267] Messrs. Scott[268] and Beheal [Vigil] arrive today with my clothes.

Sat 13. Was called on by my friend Dn. Salvadore who having heard of my resentment for the unwarrantable reasons expressed by the board of Alcaldies in regard to my charity to the Poor and tells me to not regard them and he will interfere in my behalf.

Sund 14. Attended church this morning. Visit my patients in the afternoon. Day fine.

Mond. 15. Witnessed a tumbling exhibition this evening but of an inferior Gust.[269] Patients all succeeding.

Tues. 16. Visited the temple this afternoon with Mr. Scott. Also ascended the steeple of the church which is truly a stupendous structure.[270]

Wed 17. Nothing of importance.

Thursday 18. Discharged three of venerial Patients today.

Frid 19. Several new patients under fever. Beginning to be warm and sultry.

Sat. 20. Attended church this afternoon. Had 6 or 8 calls after night, busy until 1 Ock.

---

[267]Ayuntamiento.

[268]On a list dated July 13, 1825, of trail traders who paid duties at the Santa Fe customhouse, Wm. R. Seatt [Scott] from Columbia, Missouri, provided an invoice dated March 8, 1825. Dr. Willard states that Mr. William Scott returned to Chihuahua on January 1, 1827. A few years later William Scott and his servant were issued a passport on September 25, 1830, to enter the states of Chihuahua and Sonora on commercial business. Weber, *Extranjeros*, 18, 24.

[269]"Gust" in this context apparently refers to the distance, force, and/or velocity of the apparent acrobatic performance.

[270]While the building and its architecture provide a very impressive site, its position as the tallest building between Durango, Mexico, and Saint Louis, Missouri, meant that many people were also impressed by the view.

Sund 21. May. Attended church this morning. Sermon delvd. by El Padery Baca.[271] Visited 12 or 13 patients today besides prescribing for many of the poor in the streets. Almost every day is commemorate to some Saint.[272]

Monday 22.[273] This is a day commemorated by the Heathen Christians and is Spent in visiting an old temple.[274] Fel in with the crowd. Attended a fandango in the evening.

Tues 23. This day is also commemorated as yesterday,[275] took a ride on horseback for exercise.

Wed 24. Much preparation is making for tomorrow by erecting a high Bowery around the public Square.

Thus. 25. Attended Church this morning after wich a rabble procession was formed and marched around the square occasionally kneeling to their images.[276]

Frid 26. Nothing of importance transpires.

Sat 27. May. Several patients under fever but convalescent. Illuminate this evening in front of the Church.

Sund 28. Was called in consultation in case of fever with Dr. Lopus [Lopez] who acceded to my prescription.

Mond 29. Had a call from P. Priest now at St. Diego[277] to pay him a visit if possible, but my patients here would not consent therefore declined.

---

[271]Padre Juan José Baca heard the confession of Miguel Hidalgo y Costilla, who was executed in July 1811.

[272]May 21, 1826, was the Catholic feast day dedicated to the Holy Trinity.

[273]May 22 is dedicated to Saint Rita in the modern Catholic calendar.

[274]It would make sense if the "old temple" refers to the Capilla de Santa Rita, which would then have been a short distance southwest of the town.

[275]The fiesta continues.

[276]Thursday, May 25, 1826, was the Catholic feast of Corpus Christi.

[277]These are the hot springs at San Diego de Alcalá.

Tues. 30. Write to my Father Dr. S[eth] Millington & Mr. Anderson[278] by John Vigil.

Wed. 31. Several patients from St. Pablo[279] as much business as I can attend to.

Thurs. 1 June. This is a feast day called Corpus Christus.[280] A procession was formed today.

Thus. 1st. June 1826.[281] Another procession today. My patients increase in number. Several labouring under fever.

Frid 2. Nothing of importance.

Sat. 3. Several under fever. The Virgin Mary is carried out every night and then back. Priests in the day to heal the sick.[282] But I believe without effect.

Sund 4. Have as much business as I can attend to.

Mond 5. Now most of my patients convalescent.

Tues. 6. Nothing of importance.

Wed 7. Slight shower this evening. Bevers visits today.

Thus 8. Lost an important patient last night, Don Pedro Enero who died of Pneumonia.

Frid. 9. Nothing of importance.

---

[278]Dr. Willard wrote to William Anderson in Santa Fe. Paul and William Anderson, who were identified as merchants in Saint Louis in 1818–19, formed a trading company with James Baird and others on July 23, 1822, and undertook their first trading trip across the plains. William Anderson is listed as paying the 15 percent importation duty and 3 percent excise tax on April 20, 1825. Julian [William] Anderson is listed as a merchant with a passport from his government and living in Santa Fe in Governor Narbona's monthly report of foreigners. William Anderson is also listed as leaving Taos for Missouri on April 6, 1827. Weber, *Taos Trappers*, 60–63; Weber, *Extranjeros*, 15–17, 20–21, 29–33, 36–37.

[279]Today San Pablo is known as Meoqui, which lies about 80 km (50 miles) southeast of Chihuahua.

[280]Thursday, May 25, 1826, was dedicated to Corpus Christi and Friday, June 2, 1826, was dedicated to the Sacred Heart of Jesus.

[281]Willard wrote two entries for Thursday, June 1, 1826.

[282]One of a priest's many functions is to pray for the sick.

Sat 10. But few patients at present.

Sund 11. Weather quite warm.

Mond 12. Saw a letter from Mexico stating that Government has consented to remunerate Mr. Robt. McKnight for goods confiscated before the change of government.

Tues 13. Nothing of importance.

Wed 14. Dn. Juan B. Vigil left this afternoon for N Mexico. Send by him letters to my Father,[283] Dr. Millington, Col. Storrs & William Anderson—Mr. Scott also sends letters.

Thus 15. My patients are convelesent. Weather exceedingly warm.

Frid 16. Nothing of importance.

Sat. 17. Do Do Do.

Sund 18. Discharged several patients today. Visited Col Arzas in the evening. Treated with much respect.

Mond. 19. But few patients at present.

Tues 20. Nothing of importance.

Wed 21. Feel rather indisposed. Draw off a list of medicines for Dn. Salvadore who wishes to send to Mexico [City] for a general assortment of drugs.

Thurs. 22. Sundry patients today, several from Pueblos 50 miles distant.

Frid. 23. Nothing of importance.

Satd. 24. This day is comorated to St. John the Baptist by resident to and from an old Church called by the same name. Three or four horses offered to pass the day in riding. Accept.

Sund 25. June. Patients convelesent. Visited Col Arzas family in evening.

---

[283]"Josiah Willard of New York Ancestry," www.familysearch.org/eng/search/IGI/individual_ record (accessed November 12, 2009).

Mond 26. Rode out morning & evening. From presure of business a few days past became somewhat indisposed, but much better today.

Tues. 27. Called today to see a woman who has been under the Sps Drs[284] hands a year taking medicine for the venerial and wishes other remedies.

Wed. 28. A light shower last night and today. Air cool and pleasant. Bathed this evening in the river.

Thus. 29. This day is commemorated to St. Petro.[285] Attend a play this evening. Recd. a letter from E. Standley[286] [and] another from J. Douglass at St. Fe.

Friday 30. The new Legislature convenes today. Paid the General a visit this morning who I found very polite. Many fine showers last night.

Sat. 1st July 1826. Day pleasant. Illumination last night and tonight. State officers in uniform today, to appear in which they take delight.[287]

Sund 2d. Much gambling in the public square for the day past, but more particularly today without regard to God or conscience. Made several friendly visits this afternoon.

Mond. 3. Weather pleasant. Few patients. Bathe in river this evening.

---

[284]Spanish doctors.

[285]June 29 is Saint Peter's Day.

[286]Elisha Stanley was one of the men who traveled with the packers during the 1825 spring caravan from Missouri. He apparently stayed in Santa Fe trading. Governor Narbona's February 1, 1826, report of foreigners lists "Eliseo, merchant" as a foreigner without a passport. On February 13, 1826, Stanley apparently assisted William Workman, a merchant in Taos. Workman wrote to his brother, "If it had not a been for Mr. Stanly I should have died for they was no Doctor hear and not much medisin, and it is one of the meenest Country to be sick in the world for there is no nourishment to be got." Reséndez, "Getting Cured," 89. Elisha Stanley was an experienced Santa Fe Trail trader who traveled down El Camino Real with the annual caravan from Missouri in 1826. The company of traders (size unknown) that left Fort Osage in August (1826) and reached Santa Fe in November included James Collins (at a later date, Indian affairs superintendent in New Mexico), Elisha Stanley, Solomon Houck, Edwin M. Ryland, James Fielding, Thomas Talbott, and William Wolfskill. All these men remained in Mexico for nearly a year. Barry, *Beginning of the West*, 119, 135.

[287]It appears as if the illumination and uniforms are related to the opening of the state legislature.

Tues. 4. Nothing of Importance.

Wed. 5. An increase of patients today, two under Dropsey.

Thurs. 6. A Frenchman arrives today who claims charity as a countrymen. Not at all pleased with his account of himself. Give him his supper.

Frid. 7. Heavy shower this evening with thunder and lightning.

Sat 8. Illumination rockets and procession this evening in honor of the holy Refaelia.[288]

Sund. 9. Another procession bearing a painted image of their female saint. A shower this evening.

Mond. 10. A Frenchmen arrives today and puts up[289] with me.

Tues. 11 July. Pleasant weather. Bathed this evening.

Wed. 12. A little indisposed to day from a slight pain in breast.

Thurs 13. Bleed myself this morning. Visited a ruin in company with my two countrymen in the evening.

Frid. 14. Mr. Day Dg. [Durango] leaves this morning for Paral. Write a few lines to P. Wetmore at St. Louis Potosi. Also write a letter to E. Stanley at St. Fe.

Sat 15. Showers in the evening. Rockets and illuminations at night.

Sund 16. Showers in the evening. Display of rockets at night.

Mond 17. Nothing of importance.

Tues 18. Weather fine.

Wed 19. Operated upon a case of Staphyloma[290] by excision.

Thus. 20. Shower this evening.

---

[288]The meaning of this reference is unknown.
[289]Stays overnight or bunks.
[290]Staphyloma is a protrusion of the cornea or sclera of the eye.

Frid. 21. All my patients convelesent.

Sat 22. Shower this morning. Visited a [illegible word] for the purpose of bathing.

Sund. 23. Something indisposed today.

Mond 24. Nothing of importance.

Tues 25. This day is spent in riding to and fro. Sleigh double and treble people of every class that can raise a horse is mounted.

Wed 26. This day is also spent as yesterday. Walked out in the evening and returned in company with Col. Arzas family.

27. Sent out several a/cts[291] for colls.[292] but without success.

28. Ten new patients today under different complaints and among the rest one under furious madness.

29. Much occupied with my patients having 15 or 20 to look to every day.

Sund. 30. Nothing of importance.

Mond 31. Four new patients today.

Tues 1st Augt. All of my patients convalesent. Performed Parencinteses[293] this evening, drew 1 1/2 gallons.

Augt. 2d. Set a broken arm this evening—also called up at eleven to set a broken leg.

Thurs 3. Much fatigued from visiting many patients.

Frid 4. This day introduced a new aniversary and serves to let me this eve of life comes on a year having completed 32 years.

Sat 5. Opperated upon an eye by L. Costio.

Sund 6. Wholy occupied all day in visiting patients.

[291]Abbreviation for accounts.
[292]Abbreviation for collections.
[293]Paracentesis, which is drawing fluid from the abdominal cavity. Craig Timm, M.D., email message to author, November 13, 2013.

Mond 7. Dn. Salvadore dangerously sick from a slight stroke of Apoplesy.[294]

Tues 8. All of my patients convalescent, except Dn. Salvadore.

Wed 9. Lost my good friend Dn. Salvadore this morning at 7 Ock.

Thus. 10. Attended the funeral of my good friend Dn. Salvador whose death seems to be much regretted in general.

Frid 11. Augt. Recd $12 from Priest Escontrias who in the first place refused to pay 8 the amt of my a/c. I afterwards augmented it to 12 and put it in to the hands of Sr. Cura who ordered payment.

Sat 12. Showers this evening.

Sund 13. Another small shower this evening.

Mond 14. Nothing of importance.

Tues 15. Patients all convelesent. Visit Col Arzas family in evening.

Wed. 16. Sr. Cura returns from his country seat much reduced having laboured under a diarrhea for 3 or 4 months and under a cronic Dyspepsia for several years.[295] He solicits my utmost endeavors to establish his health.

17. Nothing of much importance. Recd letter from Dn. Cozine[296] at El Passo.

18. Answered the above today.

Sat 19. Augt. Weather fine. A few showers at night.

Sund. 20. Visited patients in forenoon. Afternoon took a long walk to view the uppermost arches.[297]

---

[294]The diagnosis suggests that Don Salvador Porras was suffering from internal bleeding that generated a stroke and a possible loss of consciousness.

[295]A mercury potion was prescribed for syphilis and often resulted in mercury poisoning: indigestion, diarrhea, etc.

[296]A John H. Cozine, U.S. citizen, resided in Parral, Chihuahua, as of February 5, 1831. http://civilwarthosesurnames.blogspot.com/search?q=Cozine (accessed September 27, 2011).

[297]It is estimated that the upper arches of the colonial aqueduct are about five miles from the center of town. This aqueduct brought water from the Río Chuviscar in the west to the city. A long walk there and back would be about ten miles.

Mond. 21. Much thronged in business of my profession.

Tues 22. Nothing of importance.

Wed 23. Patients all convalesent.

Thurs. 24. Arrived yesterday two infirmed from St. Geronimo.

Frid 25. Nothing important.

Sat 26. A shower nearly every day. Recd a fine present of fruit from St. Geronimo.

Sun. 27. Heavy showers last night with heavy thunder and lightning.

Mond. 28. Much occupied with visiting patients.

Tues. 29. Weather cool and pleasant.

Wed. 30. Found Scott something indisposed. Bled him this morning.

Thus. 31. Recd. a letter from Dn. Pedro Armendaris[298] recommending his friend to me who labours under dispepsia.

Frid. 1st September 1826. Several new patients and female visits in the evening.

Sat. 2d. nothing of importance.

Sund 3d. Took a game of cards with Sr. Cura to divert him.

Mond 4. Cool & pleasant.

Tues. 5. Recd a present of an ounce of gold worth $10 from Dn. Molina.

---

[298]Don Pedro Policarpio de Azcue y Armendariz (1787–1853) was a soldier who served in the Spanish royal army at the garrisons of Chihuahua, San Elizario, and Santa Fe. Lt. Armendariz led the firing squad in the execution of Father Miguel Hidalgo y Costilla on July 30, 1811. In 1814 he retired and became a merchant in both Santa Fe and Chihuahua. In 1818 he was appointed tax collector in Santa Fe by his friend, Governor Melgares. Governor Melgares awarded him two private land grants near present-day Valverde, which resulted in Pedro Armendariz becoming one of New Mexico's largest landowners with nearly half a million acres. He went on to hold various posts in Chihuahua, including serving as magistrate of the state supreme court during the 1830s and 1840s. Almada, *Diccionario*, 46; Paul Harden, "The Pedro Armendaris Grant," *El Defensor Chieftan*, May 2, 2009, B1.

Wed 6. Called up last night by a patient from St. Cruss who came with 3 others for medical aid prescribed for them today. Hear of the death of General Boliver.[299]

Thus. 7. Nothing important.

Frid. 8. Today they commemorate the nativity of the Virgin Mary.[300] Took a walk with some friends.

Sat 9. Something indisposed from a dull pain in my back. Procession in memory of the Virgin Mary.[301]

Sund. 10. Health much better.

Mond 11. News arrives of the death of the Governor of this place who died on the 26 of last month in the City of Mexico.[302]

Tues. 12. Recd. compliments from Dn. Pedro Armendaris in Mexico [City] who is Senator from Chihuahua.

Sept. 13. 1826 Was called to a patient under Mania yesterday who still continues furiously—rain today.

Thus. 14. Rain last night and today.

Frid 15. But few patients at present except dispeptic and venerial patients.

Sat. 16. Arrived today a patient from Durango for the purpose of putting himself in care for the venerial not having confidence in the doctors there.

Sund 17. Visit my patients as usual.

Mond 18. Took home my money from Dn. Bisentes. Eleven dollars missing.

---

[299]Willard is referring to General Símon Bolívar, who did not pass away until 1830. Almada, *Gobernadores*, 10.

[300]José de Urquidi, the first governor of Chihuahua, established a fiesta dedicated to the Virgin of Guadalupe on September 8, the anniversary of the opening of the first state congress on September 8, 1824. As such, the celebration was political as much as religious. Ibid., 9.

[301]The politico-religious celebration continues.

[302]José Urquidi died in Mexico City on August 25, 1826. Almada, *Gobernadores*, 10.

Tues 19. Weather cool and pleasant.

Wed. 20. Had the curiosity today to take the dimensions of a pair of Spanish spurs which are about an ordinary size and are as follows. The bow which surrounds the heel 4 inches in diameter made heavy, carved and inlaid with silver. The rear projection containing the rowel 5 inches long. The rowel 5 inches in diameter a course chain under the foot and very wide strap over the instep. On the outside of the foot a silver plate of 3 1/2 inches diameter weighing in all I should suppose about 4 ls [pounds] cost $25.

Wed 20th Sept 1826. Mr. Scott leaves today for the mines.

Thus. 21. But few patients at present.

Frid 22. Visited the family of Dn. Pedro Olivares[303] this afternoon where I was well received.

Sat 23. Nothing of importance.

Sund 24. More patients today. Recd. presents from 2 or three Cheese from Sr. Cura a dish of Sauce & gariranses from Dn. Avellano.[304] Took chocklet at 2 places in the afternoon.

Mond 25. Called in consultation with Dr. Lopas [Lopez] in a case of colic.

Tues. 26. Collic patient much better.

Wed. 27. 8 new patients today.

Thus 28. Recd a fine present of fruit from Sr. Cura and a beautifully embroidered cravat from Dn. Jose M. Gongora.

[303]Pedro Olivares (1787–1852) was the local tax collector in Chihuahua from June 1, 1824, to August 31, 1825. He was then commissioned to supervise the collection of taxes for imported goods, or import duties. Later in life he became a merchant and lived the rest of his life in Chihuahua. Ibid., 377–78.

[304]This is Licenciado Agustín del Avellano (1791–1851). Don Agustín arrived in 1818 and continuously held innumerable positions in the state government in Chihuahua. Ibid., 52. In 1828 he purchased Hacienda de Tierra Blanca in Valle de Allende. D. P. Rose, "[Chihuahua] Haciendas around Ciudad Jimenez 1700's: Tierra Blanca," ancestry.com (accessed October 29, 2013).

Frid 29. Visited my patients this morning. Start at 1/2 past 4 for St. Geronimo. Arrive at 8 in company with J. M. Gongora, distance 7 leagues.[305]

Sat 30. Kindly recd. last night at the house of Stephen Ochoa.[306] Attended church this morning. Took a ride in coach to view the vineyards. Ball in the evening with the Priest.

Sund 1st October 1826. Return to Chiha at 12 [and] dine with Dn. Avellano. Sup with Col Arza.

Mond 2. Visited the family of Dn. Pedro Olivasis in the afternoon & took chocklet in the evening.

Tues 3. Recd. a present of gold value $21 from Dn. Pablo Guerra[307] for 3 visits.

Wed 4. Took a walk with the ladies this evening.

Thus. 5. Visit my patients as ususal.

Frid. 6. Called at 2 this morning to a case of child birth. Recd. 2 patients from Conchez[308] who put themselves under cure.

Sat. 7. An increase of patients from different parts.

Sund. 8. Recd a visit from the chiefs of the Commanch nation, was invited to dine with D Avellano but finding me unable to attend sent a varcity[309] to my room—attended the play in the evening.

---

[305]The time of departure and distance indicate an estimated speed of 6 mph, or a slow trot.

[306]Ignacio Esteban Ochoa (1808–?) is a native of Aldama who studied law in Durango and moved to Chihuahua in 1829. Almada, *Diccionario*, 372.

[307]Pablo Guerra was a native of Zuaza, Spain, and owner of the Santa Rita copper mines near present-day Silver City, New Mexico. He was a member of the Ayuntamiento de Chihuahua that supported independence and the Plan de Ayala in 1821. In March 1826 he became the equivalent of an associate justice of the state's supreme court. Ibid., 243. Upon the death of Francisco Manuel Elguea, he acted as the executor of Elguea's estate and subsequently married Elguea's widow. By this union, Guerra acquired ownership of the Santa Rita mines around 1828. In that year he was compelled by the expulsion laws to rent the mines to the newly arrived Esteban Curcier. Cosio and Anaya, *Los inmigrantes en el mundo*, 23. He was issued a passport and expelled from Chihuahua on July 19, 1828. Rangel, "Vascos en Chihuahua."

[308]Founded at the beginning of the seventeenth century, San Francisco de Conchos lies about a hundred miles southeast of the state capital.

[309]A varsity is a representative.

Mond 9. Much occupied having 20 odd patients to visit.

Tues. 10 Oct. Something indisposed today. Took Physic this morning but continued my visits as usual.

Wed 11. Feel quite ill today from the fatigue of business and medicine.

Thus 12. Weather cool & damp. Several Pheuretia[310] patients. A calamhal[311] epidemic now prevails having run through all the Southern vistiges in this governmt.

Frid. 13. Sill indisposed from catarrh.[312] Visited 20 patients & a pesant today.

Sat 14. Weather quite cool but pleasant, patients convalescent.

Sund 15. Took a ride this afternoon with three or four friends in the country.

Mond 16. Arrived this morning a caravan of mules laden with Segars.[313] No of mules 130 amt of Segars, 90.000 dollars, Medical call from St. Hermone.

Tues 17. Receipted medicines for a man in *Guahuila Texas*.[314] Cartarah

---

[310] Pleurisy.

[311] Calomel was one of the most widely prescribed drugs. The toxic mercurous chloride purge was prescribed for many illnesses such as syphilis, intestinal disorders, and cholera. Steele, *Bleed*, 323, 59, 80, 92–93. It broke down in the patient's intestine into highly poisonous components that irritated and hence acted as a powerful purgative for the bowels. Rothstein, *American Physicians*, 49–50. Therapeutically, calomel was useless, but it also contained mercury, whose toxic effects included rotting out the patient's teeth. Weber, *Mexican Frontier*, 236.

[312] Catarrh is an old word meaning inflammation of the mucous membranes, especially the airways and the nose. Steele, *Bleed*, 323.

[313] Segar is an older alternate spelling of cigar commonly used on nineteenth-century advertisements. "Cigar," http://en.wikipedia.org/wiki/Cigar (last modified November 11, 2014). Traditionally, the Spanish crown had taken over certain profitable businesses establishing royal monopolies or estancos. Spanish tobacconists are one of the oldest institutions in force in the world, with nearly four hundred years of history. They have served as an important method of tax collection for the state through the sale of the manufactured tobacco. "Estanco," http://es.wikipedia.org/wiki/Estanco (last modified August 22, 2014). See also Reséndez, "Getting Cured," 85.

[314] Coahuila is the northeastern state in Mexico on the U.S. border of Texas.

something lighter. Dined with Dn. Jose Escudero[315] & Supped with Dn. Avellano.

Wed 18. Recd. news of the death of <u>James Douglass</u>. Attended a seranade this eve.

Thus 19. Attended a Ball at Dr. J. M. Gongora. Spent the evening exceedingly agreeably.

Oct. 20. Receive many kindnesses from the people daily.

Satd. 21. But few patients at present. Spend the evening at Dña Severena.

Sund. 22. Samething indisposed.

Mond. 23. Spent the night rather ill having to rise frequently from a visitation of Diarrhea.

Tues 24. Spent the eve at Dña Seva.

Weds. 25. Spend the evening at Sr. Olivaris.

Thus. 26. But few patients. Spend most of my time in visiting my friends.

Frid 27. Mr. Standly[316] arrives today. <u>Recd 8 letters by him.</u>

Sat. 28. Visit Col. Arzas in company with friend S. Spent the eve in playing loto.[317]

Sund 29. Took a walk to the Temple & in the evening attended the Maromeros.[318]

Mond. 30. But few patients.

---

[315]José Agustín Escudero (1801–47), an attorney, was born in Parral and moved to Chihuahua in 1824. In 1825 he was elected to the city council and in February 1826 became the chief of staff of the Secretary of the State Government. In 1834 he published *Noticias Estadistica del Estado de Chihuahua*, which summarized the history and actual state of Chihuahua. It still serves as an important primary source. José Escudero went on to have a successful political career on the national scene. Almada, *Diccionario*, 192; Weber, *Taos Trappers*, 167.

[316]Elisha Stanley. See note 286.

[317]Cady, *Loto*, 10.

[318]Tightrope walkers or acrobats.

Tues 31. Spent the eve at Dña Soverenas.

Wed. 1 Nov. Nothing of importance.

Thus. 2. Weather fine & moderate.

Frid. 3 Nov. Called up last night to a woman from St. Cruis was put to bed this eve with twins.

Sat. 4. Nothing of importance.

Sund 5. Expect to leave in the morning for the feasts at St. Geronimo.

Mond. 6. Started at 7. Arrived at 11 where we found everything in readiness to commence the fiting [fighting] of the Bulls.[319] Staid until Thurs. 9th where we returned to Chihuaa. Fully satisfied with the barbarous sport. On our return find Messrs Moor,[320] Armstrong,[321] Ramsey and Anderson.

Frid 10. Visit all of my patients today having had several new calls.

Sat 11. Nothing of importance.

Sund 12. Wrote a letter to Parson [Charles S.] Robinson by Mexico [City].

Mond 13. As usual few patients.

Tues 14. Made a shuting mach with pistols. Won 3 quartillos.[322]

Wed. 15. Mr. Morton arrives today. Four new patients.

16. Nothing of importance.

17. Visited Miss G. Weather cool but pleasant.

---

[319]Little to nothing is known about the bullfighting tradition in Aldama.

[320]Vincent Moore, rather than "Moor," was mentioned in the 1831 census of American merchants in Parral.

[321]George Armstrong (1791–1850) is listed with the Spanish name of Brazo Fuerte [Armstrong] on the Report of Foreigners by Antonio Narbona, Santa Fe, February 1, 1826. His business occupation is listed as hunter and he is without a passport. On September 17, 1826, guía #17 was issued to and signed for by George Armstrong. Weber, *Extranjeros*, 21, 31 n. 15. When he died he was buried in Westport, Oldham County, Kentucky. Find a Grave Index, 1776–2012, ancestry.com (accessed November 11, 2013).

[322]A cuartillo is both the smallest silver coin, worth 1/4 of a *real*, and a liquid measure equivalent to about 1.15 liters.

18. Nothing new.

Sund. Nov. 19. Attended Ball at night at particular risqat.[323]

Mond. 20. Several pleasant visits.

Tues. 21. Several patients on my hands under variety of diseases.

Wed 22. Weather unpleasant.

Thus. 23. Recd. $24 from Cordivo for services rendered at Taos.

Frid. 24. Spent the evening at Dña Sovrn. Last night at the same of Loterilla.

Sat 25. A light shower this evening.

Sund. 26. Nothing of importance.

Mond 27. Several new patients.

Tues 28. A new patient from St. Pablo.

Wed 29. Came a patient from Parral to put himself under cure for the vel.[324]

30. Nothing of importance.

Frid. Dec. 1, 1826. Something indisposed from pain in side.

Sat 2. Health better, spent the eve at Col Arzas in comp with Mr. Stanley.

Sund 3. Vis[ited] Bissetes in compn with several ladies and gentlemen.

Mond 4. Nothing of importance.

Thus 5. A patient arrives from Incinas [Encinillas].

Wed. 6. Weather cold.

Thus. 7. Cond. curing a Priest for venel.

Frid 8. Spent the eve at Col Arzas.

---

[323]Risqué.
[324]Venereal disease.

Sat. 9 Dec. Arrived a family from Insinellas for medical aid.

Sund. 10. Presented with $20 for four visits. Dined with Sr. Olivaris at a dinner given to a few friends. Mr. Folly[325] arrives today.

Mond 11. Nothing of importance save Col. McClure & Mr. Knox arrived today and put up with me.[326]

Tues 12. This is the anniversary of the Guadelope.[327] Attended the ceremony.

Wed 13. Dr. Akins arrives today. Spend the eve at Dña Severenas.

Thus 14. Divert ourselves in several ways.

Frid. 15. Nothing of importance.

Sat 16. Visited the Secty. of State[328] with Col. McClure where we were treated with distinguished politeness.

Sund. 17. Weather fine & warm.

Mond. 18. Spent the eve at Col Arzes.

Tues. 19. Divert ourselves a quotis.[329]

Wed. Female vis in the evening.

---

[325]Mr. Henry Foley was identified as an American merchant in Chihuahua between 1837 and 1839. Enriquez y Foley [Henry E. Foley] received guía #20 on September 3, 1828. Weber, *Extranjeros*, 34. Henry Foley had a land patent issued to him on August 10, 1849, for forty acres he purchased with cash on April 24, 1820. "General Land Office Records," U.S. Department of the Interior, Bureau of Land Management, http://www.glorecords.blm.gov/default.aspx (accessed August 1, 2014).

[326]Colonel Samuel McClure (1787–1870) was born in Kentucky. A letter sent to Colonel Marmaduke from Samuel McClure states that McClure arrived in Santa Fe on August 16, 1826. McClure conducted business with former governor Baca who lived near Tomé, New Mexico. Sappington Papers, Missouri Historical Society. McClure received factura #26 and Thomas Konr factura #27 in December 1826. Given Dr. Willard's diary entry of December 11, the last name of Konr seems to be Knox. Weber, *Extranjeros*, 28.

[327]The twelfth of December is Mexico's most important religious holiday in honor of Our Lady of Guadalupe.

[328]It seems as if Dr. Willard is referring to José Augustín Escudero, secretary of state.

[329]Willard means "quoits." The game dates back to ancient Greece using rings made of rope, metal, or leather thrown over spikes. The American version of quoits is called horseshoes.

Thus 20.[330] Patients all convelesent. Had a game at quiots this afternoon.

   Case of Obstetrics at night.

Frid 22 of Dec. Nothing of importance. Attend a fandango at night.

Sat 23. Same routine of practice.

Sund 24. Mass at 12 Ock at night.

Mond 25. Paisanos give a fandango this night.

Tues 26. Cool & cloudy.

Wed 27. Many patients and many diseases.

Thus 28. Nothing important.

Frid 29. Mr. Stanley leaves this morning for N. Mexico in comp. with Mr. Anderson.

Sat. 30. Weather raw and cloudy.

Sund 31. A violent headache today.

Mond. 1st Jan. 1827. William Scott returns today.[331]

Tues 2. Attended a ball last night. Spent the eve at Col. Arzas.

Wed 3. Samething indisposed Messr &c.

Thus. 4. Do do do.

Frid 5. Do do do.

Sat 6. Health much improved.

Sund 7. Leave Chia. for St. Heronimo in Comp with Col. McClure & Scott where I visited many patients treated exceedingly polite. Returned on Tuesday weather stormy.

Wed 10. Snowed last night and this evening.

---

[330]This date should read December 21, 1826.

[331]It seems as if Mr. Scott was returning to Chihuahua from the mines rather than from the north.

Thus 11. My Amn. friends determined the isue of this horse rase by realizing \$1,022. Won myself 100 supposed to have been bet \$4,000 in all. Invited all of my friends at night to eat and drink. Most of them merry.

Frid 12. Nothing new.

Sat 13. Weather fine but Cold.

Sund 14. Pleasant.

Mond 15. Another race today for \$20 Ams. lost.

Tues. 16. Dared several debtors.

Wed. 17. Visited the temple this evening.

Thus 18. Nothing of importance.

Frid 19. Performed castration[332] today.

Sat 20. Two Ams. & one Frenchmen [Curcier written in pencil later] arrive with two wagons from St. Antonio.

❧   ☙

EDITOR'S NOTES: The first diary ends abruptly in the middle of January 1827 after the horserace in Chihuahua.

Another foreigner, Lt. Robert William Hale Hardy, an Englishman, traveled in Mexico and wrote a travel book titled *Travels in the interior of Mexico, in 1825, 1826, 1827 and 1828*. It was published in London in 1829. From Hardy's *Travels* we know he arrived in Chihuahua on April 19, 1827, and departed eight days later, on April 28. Lt. Hardy met Dr. Willard and states in his travel book, "I met an American gentleman of the name of Roland Willan, who practiced as a doctor in Chihuahua, and was very civil. He introduced me to some pleasant families, and to a French gentleman of the name of Coussier, who had lately arrived from New Orleans, by the way of Santa Rosa [Rita], the only mine, I believe, in the province of Texas."[333]

---

[332] Assume Dr. Willard was removing a tumor by castration.
[333] Hardy, *Travels*, 474–78.

Diary 2

August 12, 1827–May 18, 1828

We accordingly parted at one crossed the river and before Sta. Rosalia a league and encamped in open plains.

Sund [August] 12. [1827]. Night and morning fine. Three or four mules missing. Start at 7 [and] turned out at Salcedos Ranch middle of day. Reached Rio Parral at 10 Ock at night much fatigued.

Mond 13. Start late this morning. Arrived at El Valla de St. Bartolome after dark in camp among the Alirnors.[1]

Tues. 14. Mr. Shatzell[2] had a horse stolen last night. Suspect a young man to be guilty. Try him before the Alcalda but was aquitted. Recd. many visits from my friends or acquaintances.

Wed. 15. Was beset today by several citizens to remain a few months with them offering me two thousand dolls. in two months. I at length

---

[1] *Arrieros* is the Spanish word for muleteers.

[2] Juan Pedro Shatzell (1781–?) was born in Germany. A commercial merchant from Kentucky, he filed a declaration of intent for American citizenship on October 13, 1806. As a forty-five-year-old single man he came with Curcier and four other Frenchmen to Chihuahua in 1826. Cosio and Anaya, *Los inmigrantes*, 17–18. "Philadelphia 1789–1880 Naturalization Records," ancestry.com (accessed October 20, 2011). By 1845 he was the resident American consul in Matamoros. He claimed that his annual income as a merchant amounted to $250,000. Graf, *Economic History*, 160.

concluded to stay. Mr. Statzell leaves at 1 P.M. Visit my landlords [illegible name] in the evening who pays me great attention.

Thus 16. Recd. number of visiters today, the most of them soliciting medical aid. Defer their calls until tomorrow.

Frid. 17. D. Manuel Moreno[3] agrees to find me a house today if I am not suited with his, the best part of which he offers me, but believing it would incomode him feel a delicacy in receiving it. But agree to accept it for the present, and open my medicines. Rode out in the eve.g.

Sat 18. Visited by my friend D. Luis Porras who offers me his house which is more commodious than the one I now occupy, but on proposing a removal my lanlord opposes it no doubt from interested motives wishes my stay. He however having commenced the repairation of a room for my reception, would probibly be considered impolite to leave. Recd. six or eight visits in the eve.

Sund. 19. Attended church this morning through courtesy—walked in the evening.

Mond. 20. Opperated on a fistulae in perinio.[4] Rode out in the evening.

Tues 21. Hunted rabbits this evening. Killed one. But few patients yet spend most of my time in reading.

Wed. 22. Rode out this evening. Receive many presents of fruit from the people who manifest much courtesy.

Thurs. 23. Nothing of importance.

---

[3]Dr. Willard might not have remembered Don Moreno's first name, or perhaps Manuel was a Moreno relative. José Francisco Moreno (1789–?) was issued a passport on February 6, 1828, as one of the many Spaniards expelled from Chihuahua. Subsequently he departed from the port of Veracruz and traveled on the ship named *Monk* arriving in New Orleans on March 19, 1829, when he was forty years old. "New Orleans Passenger Lists, 1820–1945," ancestry.com (accessed October 21, 2011); Rangel, "Vascos en Chihuahua."
[4]Perinea.

Sun 26. Joseph Payne arrives today from N. Orleans, puts up with me.

Mond. 27. Start this morning with Mr. Payne for Parral, arrive at 12. Put up with the president D. Franco. Baca,[5] treated very politely.

Tues 28. Return to El. Valla.

Wed 29. Mr. Payne leaves him for Guagoquilla with expectations of returning here with goods.

[In this diary, Dr. Willard's daily activities are not recorded for the months of September–December 1827. From his autobiography we learn that he was traveling with friends and visiting over the Christmas holidays.]

Chihuahua January 22, 1828. Started at 12 ock travel? 20 miles. Night cold.

W. 23. My horse breaks loose and runs off. Send 2 servants in pursuit of him and proceed 2 leages for water and encamp for to wait my servants return.

Th? 24. Dispach another servant for Dolores expecting my horse may have gone there.

Fri 25. Two srvts return from Chihua. without success. Mr. Storrs having arrived dispaches letters from the U. States to me.

26. Leave the spring this afternoon & was overtaken by a man who brings my horse. Pay him $4 for his trouble. Arrive at St. Pablo distance 60 ms. from Chia; here I bought a horse and mule, the former for $7 and the latter for $12 in clothes.

Sund 27. Leave St. Pablo and travl to bend of river Conchez dis 25 ms.

Mond. 28. Traveled to D. Anto [Antonio] Palacios [H]acienda dis. 14 ms.

Tues 29. Mr. Shatzell arrived at my lodgings last night from Veracruz.

---

[5]President of municipal council of Parral, Mexico.

Started at 8. Traveled 25 ms. & encamped without water. Passed Sta. Rosalia at 12 ock distance from St. Pablo 50 ms.

Wed. 30. Started this morning at 8. Got to water at noon. In crossing the ditch 2 mules mired [and] had some trouble in getting them out. Traveled 24 ms. Encamped without water.

Thus. 31. One horse missing this morning belonging to Mr. F. Send a man back in pursuit of him. We proceed to the ranch of D. J. M. Abellano. Decd dis 11 ms. Man returns without the horse. Concluded to stay all night where we were kindly entertained by the old lady who also furnished us with provisions of all kinds, to last us to Mappimi, and would receive no compensation whatever.

Friday 1st February [1828]. Passed to day Agusts [Augusto] Corderos ranch ocupied by his brother who solicited me to light and stay to breakfast. Consented. Travelled 25 ms. Encamped without water.

Sat. 2. Traveled 20 ms. Passed Las Canas [Canoas] 4 leagues & encamped without water.

Sund. 3. Was overtaken by two ruffians whom had before sold us a mule & horse in St. Pablo. They asked leave to stay with us overnight which we granted. About an hour before day they arrose and put off with all my small clothes. Missed them at sunrise. Pursued them as I supposed for 12 miles without success. Passed St. Blass and St. Bernardo. Distance from last nights encampment 27 [miles].

Mond. 4. Passed Andaras and encamped within 3 leagues of Pelayo where we encamped without water.

Tues 5. Arrived at Pelayo at 10 ock. We conclude to remain until tomorrow.

Wed. 6. Start this morning at 1/4 after 9. Passed a pond of water & encamped at 1/2 past 3. Traveled 14 ms.

Thus 7. Another accident last night more serious than ever, my best horse having been stolen between 7 & 8 while standing tied within

40 yards of our beds. Knowing him to be stolen, make no search. Start at 1/2 after 7 [and] arrive at 1/4 of 5 at Mapimi much fatigued. Distance 25 ms.

Frid 8. Spend this day endeavouring to git another servant and animals but without success. Mapimi is a small filthy villiage containing 8 smelting furnaces all worked by the Europeans which are about leaving for the U.S. The whole country manifests extreme poverty.

Sat. 9 Feb. Started from Mapimi at 11. Proceeded to the well 14 ms. Here we had to pay for watering the beasts.

Sund 10. Started late this morning. Arrived at the river Nasas at 3 which we found high. Here the ferry men asked $6 pr. load, paid him 4 & swam the beasts. A terible wind arrose which filled the air with sand. We urged on to get to grass, but night overtaking us before we got out of the woods & were obliged to tie the animals by the head all night.

Mon 11. Started early this morning and travelled until after dark without finding grass tied the beasts.

Tues. 12. Started early this morning and proceeded until 1/2 after 3 when we came to water & sent the mules a league to grass. Distance from the well 70 miles.

Wed 13 Feb. Conclude to remain here today to rest the beasts which are much reduced for want of food.

Thurs. 14. Start late this morning. Arrive at St. Lorenzo at dark. Distance from Mapimi 108 ms.

Frid 15. Conclude to spend the day at this place and feed on straw and corn. Rode up to Parras a leagues distance from this, for to buy provisions. Here the grape is cultivated to a very considerable perfection it being the principal article of commerce as they make them into wine and brandy. The farm of St. Lorenzo occupies from 150 to 200 hirelings the year round, and is owned by a young widow. The vineyard occupies something like 250 acres, and the dwelling house occupies a square of 275 feet each front and is subdivided into 4 squares by a chain of rooms running through the centers at right angles the whole finished in good stile.

The out buildings are numerous besides the houses of the peasants which form a very considerable villiage constituting a population of about 600 souls. [in pencil the following phrase is inserted: "all owned by a widow"]

Sat. 16. Started this morning at 1/2 8. Arrived at Pata galona dis 21 ms. Here we bought corn for the animals at 3.75 finega[6] and paid 25 cts. for water.

Sund 17. Feb. Our travel today was over rocky hills and crooked roads. Arrived at a small ranch called Macuyu, distance 20 ms.

Mond. 18. Passed de Acienda called Patos. Here the director of the English plantations resides, who urged us hard to tarry until the morrow but conclude to proceed to a small ranch called Mimbre, distance from Parras 60 ms.

Tues 19. Arrive at Saltillo at dark after passing an exceedingly bad road, having travelled 25 ms. This place is of considerable importance containing some 10 thousand inhabitants, including the Indian population, which constitutes a large portion of the population and who appear to live in very comfortable sircumstances, their habitacions abounding with fruits and virdure.

The stile of building here is far superior to that of Chihua. with paved streets &c. It is said that Mr. Bearing and sons owns all the land laying between the place and Parras for which he is to pay a little short of $1,000,000 but has pd but $100,000 as yet, his title being in dispute.

The purchase I should think as injudicious one. As most of the land over which we passed, manifests a barren unproductive soil, but principaly for the want of water. The distance from Parras to this place is something like 85 miles, the ~~width~~ length of s. purchase I have not been able to learn tho said to be 240 miles long. The climate is something

---

[6]*Fanega* is a Spanish word for a measure of grain by volume equivalent to 1.5 bushels.

like that of Orleans, though vegetation is perhaps more forward. We were invited into the garden this morning by a very friendly Italian who has resided here some 10 or fifteen years, and who thinks Orleans more forward, but as we found flax, peas and many other things in blossom would presume he might be mistaken. The valley in which Saltillo is situated is rich and beautiful & being surrounded by ragged mountains on everyside, renders the country quite picturesque indeed. We were invited by D. Jose Rosi to dine, who set a very excellent table and treated us with politeness and hospitality. Here we found a Mr. Miller Post from N. York but a Frenchman by birth, who is here merchandizing.

Wed 20. Conclude to spend the day in this place having found 3 or 4 Ams. all of which are on the point of leaving.

Thurs. 21. Start at 1/2 past eleven [and] arrive at Ojo Caliente at dusk dis. 18 ms. This day we passed many fine farms, and beautiful country. We passed a continuous full stone wall of at least 3 miles in length and strait as a line. This wall enclosed a piece of wheat of 1,000 acres at a moderate calculation which looked exceedingly well. Close by this field we paid 75 cts pr wt. of straw and $6 pr. finega for corn & 25 cts. for room.

Frid 22 Feb. Proceeded as far as the Rinconada. Arrived at middle of the day, distance 12 ms. Here we are obliged to stop until tomorrow as there is no food or water for the animals within 6 leagues distance from here.

Sat. 23. Start early this morning. Felt quite indisposed last night and conclude to fast this morning, taken with a colic at 10 which lasted until 2 when we arrived at Santa Catarina, distance 18 ms.

Sund 24. On inquiring find they required us to stay until after service as its considered as act of sacrilige to leave town before. We through politeness conformed. Started at 1/2 past 10. Arrived at 1/2 past 2 at Monterey, dist. 12 ms. This place contains something like 9,000 souls and tolerably well built for this country. We found here 2 or 3

Americans for whom we agree to wait as they propose accompanying us in 3 or 4 days to Refugio.[7]

Mond. 25. The church in this place is large and of tolerable arcitecture, no other buildings of note. Vegitation resembles the month of May as many shrubs are in blossom. I also saw some orange trees laden with fruit. This place manufactures a good deal of sugar from the cane and furnish all the upper country with this article.

Tues 26. Weather quite warm. Commerce appears to be very dull it being confined mostly to petty grocery keeping. The poor manifest less distress than at Chihuahua & the Valle, there being a very few in comparison, to towns west and north.

Wed. 27. Conclude to take out a guía for my money for fear of confiscation. Paid for same $35. Was visited by Genl. Gutieres[8] former governor of Tamulipas who ordered Irtibide put to death he giving me a concise account of the same. He now officiates as Col under pay of 2.713 annally and lives apparently quite inactive.

28 Feb. 1828. Nothing of importance save our Amn. servant having been in a drinking spree several days. Has at length became sober and returned to beg my pardon & wishes to go on but having fortunately assertained his future intentions to be corrupt he having communicated to another servant the bare faced plan of combining with several soldiers and the two other servants for the purpose of robing & murdering us on the road. I consequently discharged him forth with tho considerably indebt.

Frid 29. Intended starting today but the weather proving inclement and Mr. Adams concluding [to] go with us agree to stay until tomorrow.

Sat. 1st March 1828. Started this morning at 8 ock & arrived at Cadaritta[9] at 4 P.M., dis 24 mls. This place contains something like

---

[7]Governor Lucas Fernández issued a decree in 1826 that Villa del Refugio would be renamed Villa de Matamoros, to honor Mariano Matamoros, known as the hero of Mexican independence.

[8]General Juan Francisco Gutiérrez served as governor three times between September 23, 1823, and July 18, 1824.

[9]Cadereyta, Nuevo León, Mexico, founded in 1637.

3,000 souls and manifests a more industrious aspect. Their staple commodity is the raising of cane & manufacturing it into brown shugar. The art of refining has not found encouragement among them yet.

Sund. 2. We here meet two or three Frenchmen & one American. One of the Frenchmen prevails on us to tarry here a day that he may accompany us to the coast he having money to cary could not go safely alone; we consent to wait. Dined with an Italian physician today who treated me politely.

Mond 3d March. The Frenchman yet unable to start, his mules not having come, conclude to start without him, leave at 8 Ock arriving at 5 having travelled 30 miles.

Tues 4. Started this morning at 1/4 8. Arrived at 4. Traveled 22 miles and put up at a ranch called Mantaca. Nothing to be bought but corn at 4 Shs pr Alenoz.

Wed 5. Discharged a servant this morning who urged his services for his board and conveyance but fearing his intentions were evil gave him 4 shillings to buy his provisions with orders not to show his face now. Arrived at Caggos, dis 18 ms.

Thurs 6. Mssrs Day of Duran[go] & D. Pedro arrive last evening late. Conclude to start early this morning. Accordingly arrose at 5. Start at 1/2 past 5 and proceed to Camargo,[10] distance 33 miles. Here we send the animals to a cornfield.

Frid 7. Proceed to a small ranch where neither food for man nor beasts could be had at any price. Distance 25 miles.

Sat. 8. Started at 4 [and] proceeded to Renosa[11] where we passed the heat of the day. Got a little corn at 5 shilings pr. aleno[z]. Proceed on to another ranch where we found grass for the first time since leaving Mappimi. Traveled this day 35 Ms.

Sund 9. Proceed on and encamp in open prairie. Keep a watch all night. Dis 30 Ms.

---

[10]Camargo, Tamaulipas, Mexico, founded in 1749.
[11]Reynosa, Tamaulipas, Mexico, founded in 1749.

Mond 10. Started at 1/2 after 4 and arrived at the villiage of Matamoras at 10 ock. Presented our guias to the customhouse which passed without examination of packs. Dis 12 Miles.

Tues 11. Started this evening for the ranch of Palo Blanco with my beasts, distance 30 miles, where I arrived the next morning at 9 ock. Returned to town again in the evening much fatigued.

Wed 12. Spend the day loungering.

Sunday 30th. March. Since my last minutes, not much of importance has transpired having spent my time rather idley. I however visited the coast last week which is a fine harbor but a bad enterance. There were five vessels mostly from Orleans and a Brig & Sloop men of war laying off near the harbour. Consul Smith,[12] 2 other friends and myself smuggled down $900 which I placed in the hands of Capt. Savage for safe keeping. [In pencil is written *Note arrive at coast suppose Gulf of Mexico*] Matamoras is said to contain 8 or 9,000 inhabitants but in a manner all poor living in shanties made of cane.

There are 6 or 8 good houses of brick owned by Americans & French. The principal merchants are Godfrey,[13] Lord, Smith, Cutter,

---

[12]Daniel W.[illard] Smith, originally from Connecticut, moved to Matamoros in 1821, where he served as the "unofficial consul" for some time before officials in Ciudad Victoria wrote to the Matamoros mayor as early as 1823 that they did not want him as the American consul there. Melisa Galvan, email message to author, November 4, 2013. Smith was appointed by President Monroe at the request of thirty-four New Orleans firms engaged in shipping at Refugio (now Matamoros). Smith served as U.S. consul in Refugio from 1825 to 1832 and Matamoros from 1832 to 1842. According to Graf, Smith was "well versed in the peculiarities of the trade and skillful in coping with the idiosyncrasies of the Mexican bureaucracy." Graf, *Economic History*,160; Walter B. Smith II, *America's Diplomats*, 219; Chauncey Devereux Stillman, *Charles Stillman, 1810–1875* (New York, 1856), 5–8.

[13]Benjamin Godfrey (1794–1862) was born in Chatham, Massachusetts, and served in the War of 1812 as a seaman in the gunboat flotilla. Godfrey first shows up in the Matamoros municipal archives in 1823. He and William Moore solicited permission from the local authorities to sell various items that were imported from New Orleans. Godfrey had a documented case of a shipwreck in 1824 as master of the brig *Inteligencia*, which fell victim to the sandbar at the Brazos de Santiago. He met with customs officials in Refugio to have his damages assessed and a report was transmitted to the town of Padilla. Interestingly, the port had yet to open officially to foreign commerce at that time. As a New Orleans shipping merchant at Matamoros, he made a fortune before settling in Alton, Illinois, in 1833. He died there in 1862.

& Tannier, Hale,[14] LaFon,[15] Dr. Bowers, Divine, Pendergrass[16] and others.[17] There are several houses going up mostly of brick, which are made here; all lumber is brought from the States. Provisions of all kinds are scarce and dear! Board is worth a dollar pr. day or $20 pr. month.

The American caracter is rather depreciated from the abuse of certain libertines who escape to this place as a retreat from justice that awaited them in the U.S. from whence they came. A house was broken open last week and robed of $800. A part of the same was found with a Mr. Cope, butcher in this place, who was apprehended but persisted in declaring himself innocent of the charge. He was however permitted to be taken out by the Ams. who led him into the woods where he confessed the charge and disclosed the consealment of the balance of the money and now remains for a further trial.

Sat. 12th. Apr. Brasas St. Iago.[18] Arrived here day before yesterday hoping to embark shortly for N. Orleans. The prospect however is bad, as the water on the bar is exceedingly shoal there being from 5 to 6 feet. The last week sold my mules @ $23 each, one horse @ 25 [and] another @ 10. Pack saddles at Cost fix.[19] Left Matamoras on Wednesday last with all my effects and cash $1,500 of which I succeeded in smugling and 900 prior making $2,400 saving $84 which is the amt. of duties.

---

[14]Thomas Hale was a merchant who sued Francisco Cantu for not following through on a contract to transport twenty-four boxes of clothing to Monterrey and Saltillo in 1836.

[15]Ramon LaFon (1791–1832) was born in Coutras, France. He immigrated to the United States arriving in New Orleans on May 16, 1823. He arrived in Refugio later in 1823. As a maritime merchant he was caught multiple times by Mexican authorities smuggling tobacco and dry goods into the country from New Orleans. He operated a number of different schooner vessels, trading goods with locals in exchange for Mexican silver. He was murdered in Matamoros in 1832 and buried in a crypt of the Sagrado Corazon Church in Matamoros. "Message Boards—Ramon LaFon," ancestrylibrary.com (accessed October 18, 2013).

[16]Benjamin Pendergrass (1797–1847) was born in Buncombe County, North Carolina, and died in Matamoros in 1847. Pendergrass family tree, http://www.tribalpages.com/tribe/familytree?uid=reenie155&surname=Pendergrass (accessed October 6, 2013).

[17]By 1832, three hundred foreigners were living in Matamoros, the majority of them merchants. The bulk of this Mexican trade went through New Orleans on U.S. ships. Alonzo, *Tejano Legacy*, 71.

[18]Brazos Santiago was a Mexican port of entry. Today it is called Port Isabel, Texas.

[19]On January 22, 1828, Dr. Willard paid $22 for saddles in Chihuahua, according to his account book. See appendix 2.

Wed. 15. Day before yesterday we attempted to get out of this port but all our exertions proved abortive. We however got out but the wind and waves being against us was driven back onto what is called the north brakers on which we like to have lost the vessel, but through unrestricted exertions got into harbour again. Yesterday the wind continued ahead and today so much invelloped in fog that rendered it unsafe to attempt it.

Thurs 16. Sent the pilot over the bar this morning to examine the depth of water which he reported to be sufficiently deep. Accordingly we made trial in the evening with the assistance of several boats crews and succeeded without accident. At 6 P.M. set sails. A stiff breeze soon sprang up when we were tossed at a rate no wise tollerable. This wind lasted 2 days & 2 nights in which time I lay prostrate under the direful effects of sea sickness in its most aggravated mature, alternately exercised with the most distressful of all sickness, namely vomiting. Yesterday I attempted to leave the cabin but was unable to remain long on deck altho the sea had been over considerably calm.

Mond 21. Feel myself very sick tho convelesent with an increasing appetite. Head way yesterday & today is quite moderate with a light wind directly ahead. Today at 12 find ourselves in latitude 28 deg. 27 ms. distance some 100 or 130 miles from the Bulus.[20]

Tues. 22d. Land in sight at daylight this morning. Pilot came on board at 8 ock. Find we are at the H.M. Pass. The pilot made every exertion to enter, but proved abortive; went on shore with the Capt. & pilot where I staid all night, being well treated by the pilot & family.

Wed 23d. Was awoke at daylight this morning by the discharge of 2 steamboats which came down from Orleans having ships in too [tow], one had a Ship & Brig as the same time; at about 9 ock a breeze arrose which enabled our Schooner to enter and before I could get a man off with me, she passed a mile, where he said too for me. I however succeeded in getting on board at the expence of 10 blisters on my hands, and the boatman's fee which he took tho reluctantly. The wind continues good all day which enabled us to arrive at fort Jackson[21] at dark where

---

[20]La Balize, Louisiana.

we laid too. At eleven a very light breeze showing up we accordingly spread sail but the wind & current being ahead it was two hours before we could make the point. We however succeeded and got well under way.

Thurs. 24th. The vessel flies today as if on wings. Came to the English bend at 3 ock which obliged us to stern wing and current. At this place lay 12 vessels which were unwilling to risk a trial, as also our Captain, but the mate being ambitions prevailed, we accordingly succeeded tho the vessel was many times on its side when sudden gusts would strike the sails. The shores about 50 miles below Orleans is a continuation of fine Shugar plantations. Arrived at Orleans at 6 Ock having been 31 hours from the S.M. pass 26. actual sailing, distance 115 miles against a forceable current.

Frid 25. Commenced bourding with Mr. Sprague at 5 pr. week. Landed my trunks today [and] took my species to the U.S. Branch Bank.

Sat. 26. Exchanged my money today for U.S. paper at par. Bought a suit of clothes @ $45.25 consisting of 6 shirts 2 vests 2 pantaloons 2 pr. drawers & roundabout &c &c.

Sund 27. Took a walk up the steamboat landing this morning but find none destined to St. Louis.

Mond. 28. Visited the steam boat landing today and engage a passage to St. Louis at $30.

29. Spend most of the day in walking about town. This place displays a great deal of wealth & business. Immence quantities of cotton & shugar are shipped off dayly, the former worth 9 & 10 cts, the latter 7 & 8 pr. pound. At this time there is lying in the harbor 200 sail many of which are ships besides the steam & flatboats.

30 Wed. Was to have started today for St. Louis but the troops of which our cargo consists not being ready, are obliged to defer it until tomorrow. Visited in company with Mr. Fletcher[22] the public burying

---

[21]Fort Jackson in Louisiana was constructed from 1822 to 1832, some seventy miles from New Orleans.

[22]On July 28, 1827, Johnhun [Joshua] Fletcher, a merchant from New Hampshire, was issued guía no. 31 at the custom house in Santa Fe and was bound for Chihuahua. Weber, *Extranjeros*, 32, 41.

grounds which speaks the dolful tales of mortality until the present time. Though a flourishing City, has been a grave to thousands. Christian strangers may be here shocked with the sacraligious abuses of monuments and tooms of fallen strangers, to whose memory splendid monuments have been dedicated, and since broken and effaced in a most shocking manner. This shurely bespeaks the want of natural humanity which even warms the *savage breast.*

Like the Spanish & French nations, the Sabbath is made a day of recreation. The churches appear more an article of ornament than of use, as but few leave to go up to its solemn feasts.

May 1st. The Officers and soldiers got on board and we were under way at 10 Ock.

Sund. 4. Arrived at Natches yesterday at 5 P.M. This is a hansome place affording quite a picturesque scenery. It is well built on an elevated situation dressed in shrubbery. Here I found Mr. Marble my messmate to the Spanish Co. Cntry. At this place came on board for St. Louis Dr. McPheters,[23] Mr. Taylor, Mr. Patterson & two ladies wife & wifes sister of the Dr.

Touched at Vicksburg where we received 5 others passengers. Have now on board something like 170 passengers 145 of which are soldiers together with the military and private baggage. The officers consist of

> Col Taylor {afterwards President [written in pencil]}
> Capt. Smith
> Leiut Juett
> Leiut McKinsay
> Leiut Reynolds

Leiut Jarey all of whom appear to be very polite unassuming modest Ams. which enables us to pass the time very agreable in deed. The river overflows the whole country down to Batton Roug[24] though is now on the fall. Warrington stands under water. Viksburg is built on the side of an abrupt bluff. Spend most of the day in reading tracts &c.

---

[23]Dr. William McPheeters (?–1905) of North Carolina would become a prominent citizen of Saint Louis.
[24]Baton Rouge.

Wed. 7. Passed at 10 ock the village called Memphis which is handsomely situated on a high bluff. Yesterday we passed St. Helena at 5 Ock. Here the first highland commences on the west side of the river; thus far the lowlands have been under water for 4 weeks. We continue to run night and day [and] generally average 100 miles in 24 hours.

Thurs 8. Arrive at the mouth of Ohio at 8 Ock. Call at a small place 5 miles above the mouth called Trinity which has been under water for several weeks. Got into the upper Mississippi at 11. Found the current much more powerful. Passed Cape Girardeaux at 9 P.M. Here we took in other passengers which renders us much crowded.

Sund. 11th. Arrive at the garrison[25] this morning at 8. Rained copiously last night and this morning which much incommoded the deck passengers. Visited the garrison this morning which is beautifuly situated on a high bluff immediately on the river. At this place are several good buildings of stone [and] a brick hospital newly completed of sufficient capacity for the present number of troops. Arrived at 1 P.M. at St. Louis where I found several of old acquaintances.

Wed. 14. Leave for St. Charles this morning in company with Mr. Mack. Arrived at 3 P.M. Here I met most of my old neighbors who received me very kindly, but many have sunk to rest.

Thurs. 15. Spent the evening at the house of Mr. Hays. The next day I walked out to the farm of Dr. Seth Millington who entertained me in viewing his fields, gardens, orchards, nurseries, silkworms and other apparatus.

Sat. 16 [17]. Returned to town next morning in company with Dr. M. where we examined the condition of my house and premises finding them in tolerable repair.[26] Spent the evening at M. Pettuses in compy with Mr. Horatio Lilley.

Sund 18 May 1828. Left St. Charles this morning at 10. in the Stage for St. Louis, passing through Florisant.

---

[25]Jefferson Barracks, started in 1826, is located south of Saint Louis.

[26]Dr. Willard purchased his house on Main Street in Saint Charles, Missouri, in 1820 for $300 from Mr. and Mrs. Samuel Shaw and Charles C. Machett. Land Deed, November 26, 1820. Saint Charles Historical Society.

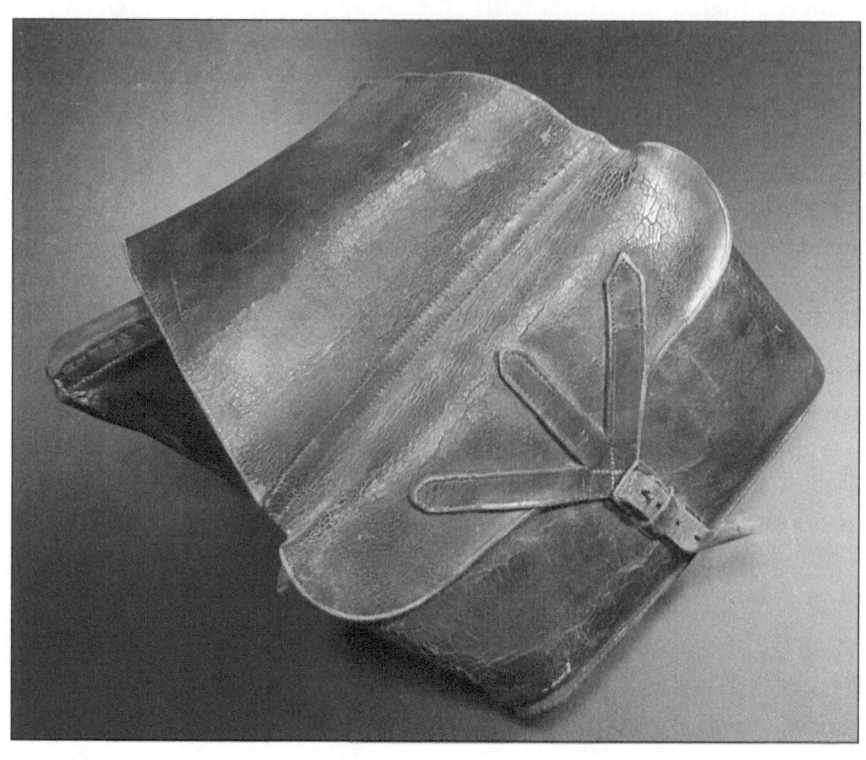

Dr. Willard's saddlebag
Descendants of Dr. Willard donated one set of his small saddlebags
to the Haddonfield Historical Society. He had sold his
larger set of saddlebags in Matamoros before
sailing home to the United States.
Courtesy of the Haddonfield Historical Society,
Haddonfield, New Jersey.

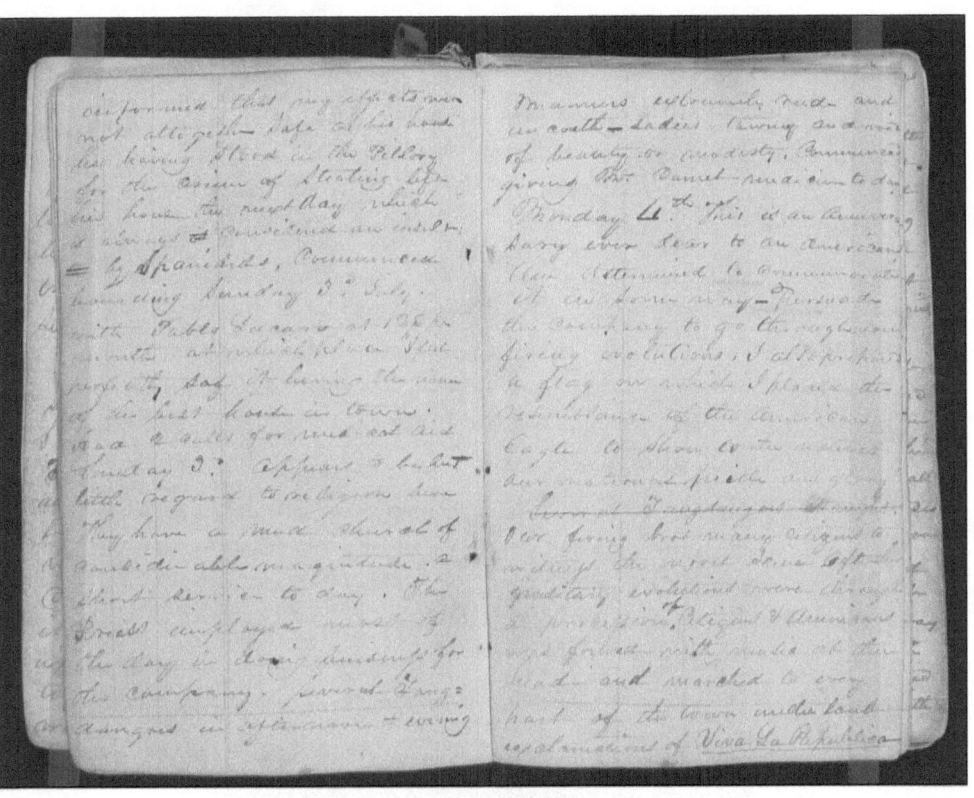

Facsimile of Rowland Willard's diary
Willard, Rowland. 1794–1884.
Unrecorded Santa Fe Trail Diary 1825–1827.
Autograph manuscript diary, 70ll. recto and verso,
8vo (4 × 6 inches). *Courtesy of the Rowland Willard and
Elizabeth S. Willard Papers, Beinecke Rare Book and
Manuscript Library, Yale University.*

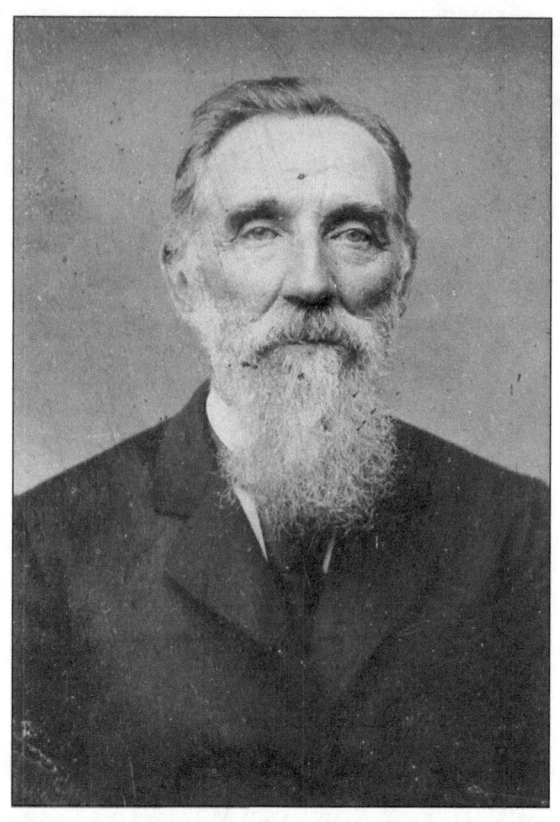

ROWLAND WILLARD AS AN ELDERLY MAN
Taken after Dr. Willard retired to Haddonfield, New Jersey, ca. 1875.
Courtesy of the Rowland Willard and Elizabeth S. Willard Papers,
Beinecke Rare Book and Manuscript Library, Yale University.

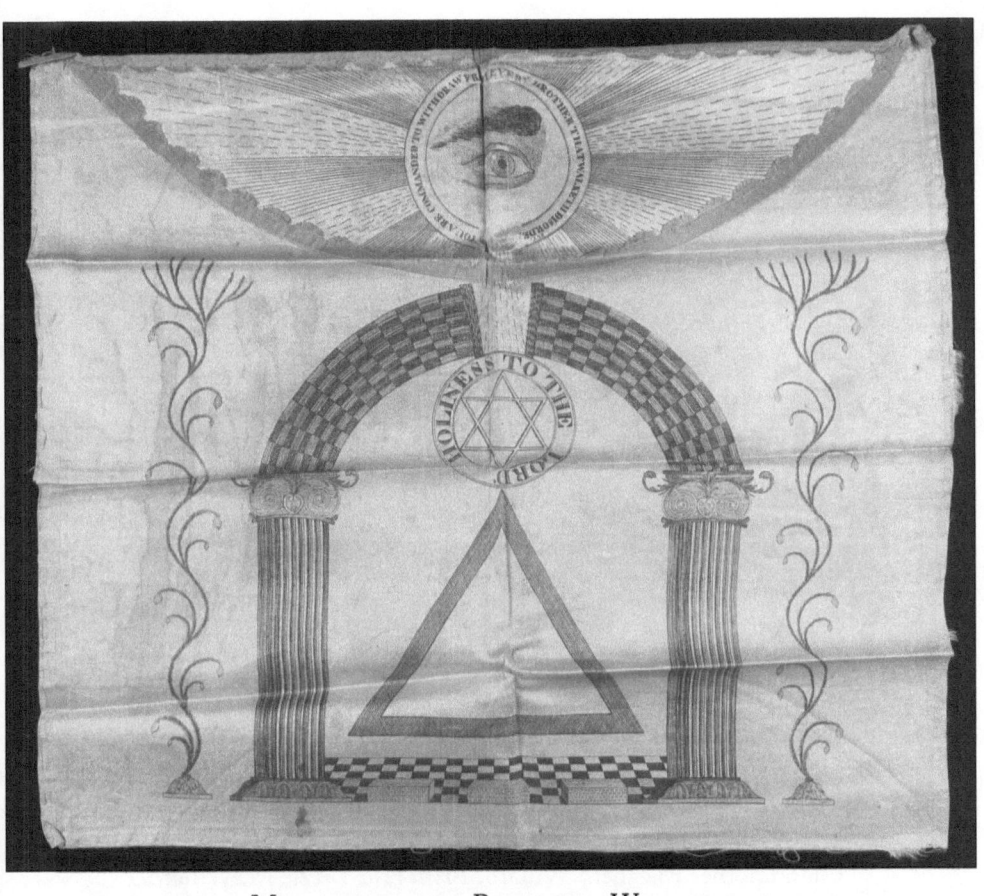

MASONIC APRON ROWLAND WILLARD
OBTAINED IN SAINT CHARLES, MISSOURI, IN 1822
He was a member of the Hiram No. 3 Lodge and served as a junior warden.
The apron features royal arch and keystone symbols of
York Rite Freemasonry. *Courtesy of the Rowland Willard and
Elizabeth S. Willard Papers, Beinecke Rare Book and
Manuscript Library, Yale University.*

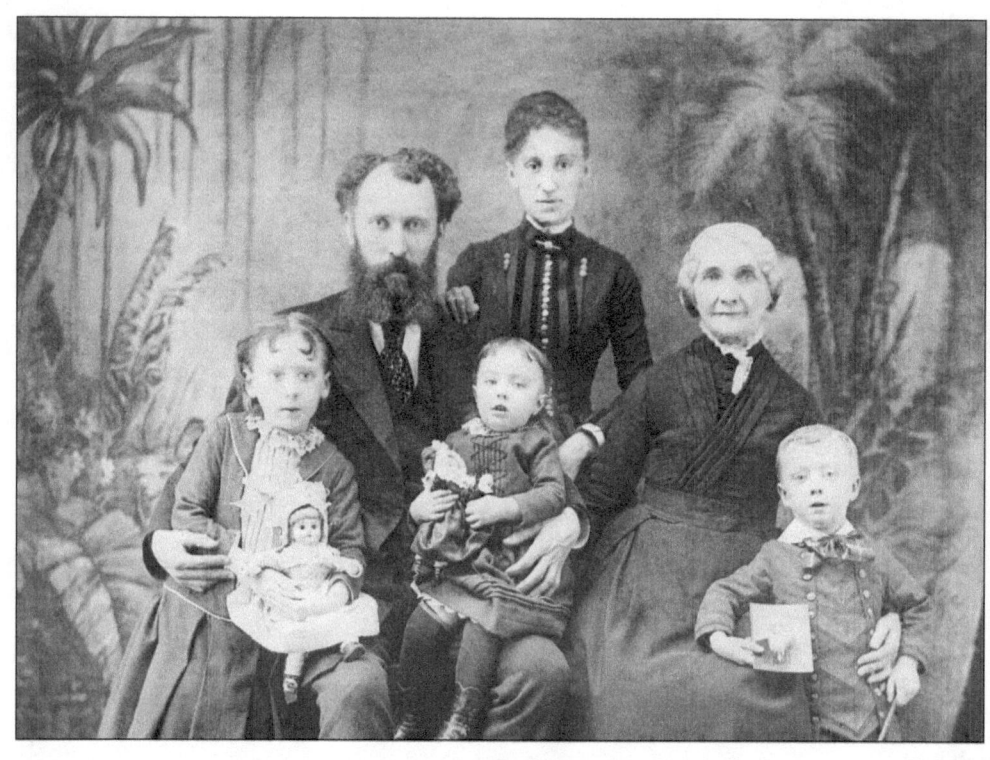

Rowland Willard, Jr., family portrait in
Haddonfield, New Jersey, taken sometime after 1885
Back row: Rowland Willard, Jr., Isabella Willard,
Grandmother Elizabeth Willard. *Front row:* Lizzie M. Willard,
Clara B. Willard, Rowland H. Willard holding a portrait of his grandfather,
Dr. Rowland Willard. *Courtesy of the Rowland Willard and Elizabeth S.
Willard Papers, Beinecke Rare Book and Manuscript
Library, Yale University.*

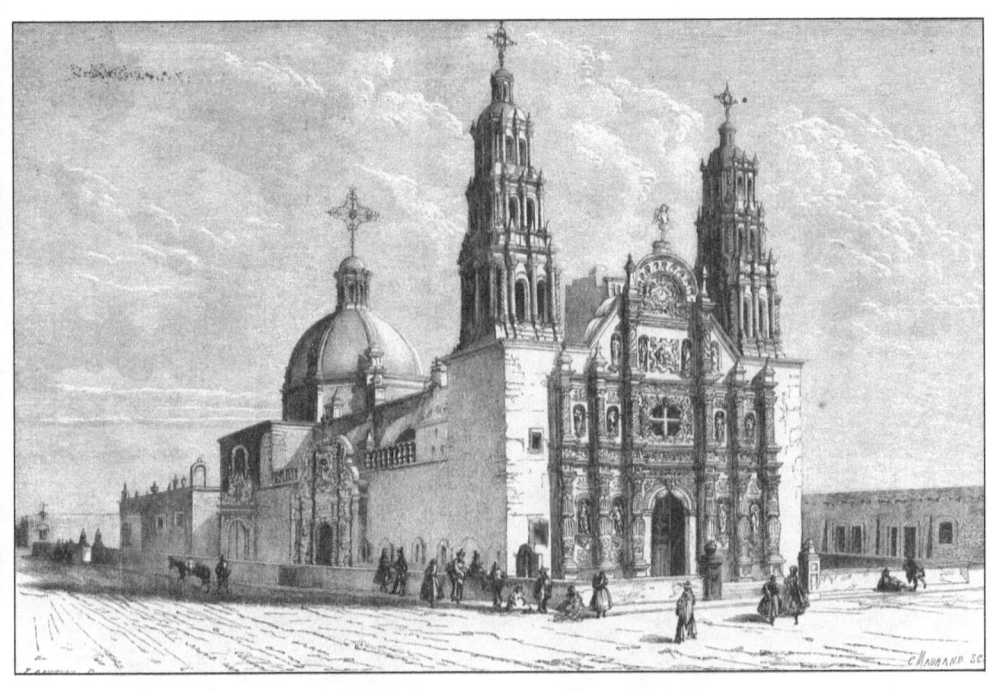

SPANISH BAROQUE CATHEDRAL ON
THE PLAZA DE ARMAS IN CHIHUAHUA, MEXICO
The cathedral was completed in 1826.
Original drawing is by Dieudonne Auguste Lancelot and
engraved by Charles Maurand, housed in the Cabinet de Estampas,
Bibliothèque nationale de France. Reproduced here from Philippe Rondé,
"Voyage dans l'état de Chihuahua (Mexique) 1849–1852,"
Le Tour de Monde (1861): 137.

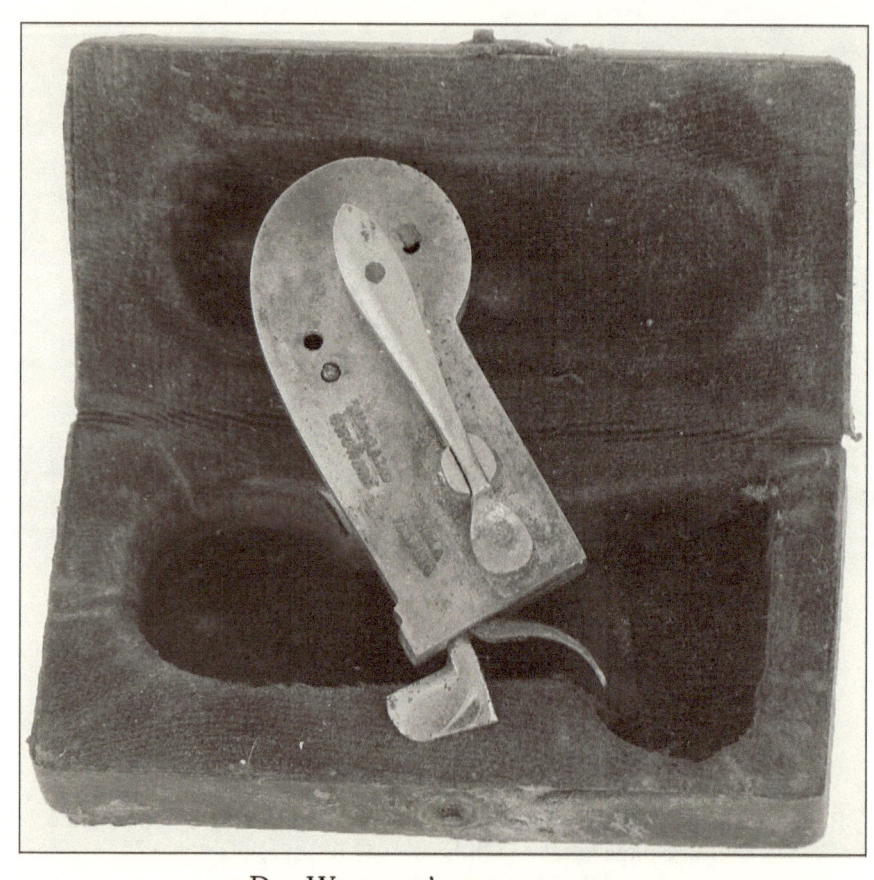

DR. WILLARD'S SCARIFICATOR
This spring lancet with carrying case served as
Dr. Willard's medical tool for phlebotomy, or bloodletting.
Photo courtesy of Nancy Mathers, a descendent of Dr. Rowland Willard.

Autobiography of
Dr. Rowland Willard

EARLY IN THE SPRING OF 1825 it was reported that quite a company of traders were fitting out for New Mexico, & were to start as soon as the spring should open. I was now tiptoe for adventure, & from what I could assertain of the country & climate (of Mexico), I suddenly made up my mind to be one of the company.[1] The intermittent fever would throw me down every few days but I nevertheless persevered in making myself ready for the expedition. I ordered two portable trunks or cases of drawers, made exceedingly light of pine, and covered with buckskin. These could be thrown open so as to form a neat display of lay billed [labeled] drawers denoting the medicines within & which I found exceedingly convenient where ever I stoped.

I purchased two good horses, saddle & Bridle with other things necessary for a long wilderness trip or journey.

The friends were very kind in rendering me any assistance in their power & were the more officious as the company had passed through town some twelve days before.

We could still hear of them however as lingering in the upper settlements, that the grass might be sufficient to subsist our animals.

---

[1]Willard would have learned about the trading expeditions to Santa Fe through word of mouth and articles published in the *Missouri Intelligencer*. In 1824 the organizing meetings were held at Shaw's Tavern, where they likely took place again in 1825, the year Willard decided to travel west.

I had a good rifle, & having ordered a brace of rifle pistols was detained for the completion.[2] All things were at length in readiness, & I set off in company with a young man by the name of Albert Boon[e][3] (a grandson of the celebrated Daniel Boone) he wishing to visit his Bro in law some four days travel on my way. My friends honored me with salutations of parting, & kindly invoked a protecting providence to accompany my process, considering it as they did, an adventure of some moment at that time.

I left St. Charles on 6th of May 1825 setting my face toward a foreign land, determined to overcome any obstacles that might impose themselves in my way, confident that with ordinary good fortune, I would make it pay something. After leaving Colonel Warners & my companion Boon, pressed forward in order to overtake my company before they should leave the settlements. The season was quite rainy, & the creeks & rivers high & some were passed with difficulty. I remember that when coming to the Sharriton,[4] I found it swimming. To swim my horses with their loads, would subject myself, clothes & medicines to injury at least if not to ruin, & I was at first at a loss how to surmount the obstacle. But having purchased a coil of small rope

---

[2]Willard used the rifled pistols he ordered from John Adams, Gunsmith, to shoot birds (such as when he went "a crowin") and other small game. John Adams of Saint Charles, Missouri, placed an advertisement in the newspaper: "GUNSMITHING—The subscriber has commenced the Gunsmithing business in a shop opposite Collier's store in St. Charles where he would keep on hand a general assortment of GUNS, and make Rifles or Fowling Pieces to suit purchasers at short notice. All kinds of repairs in the time of his business executed with dispatch. Cash paid for old brass. John Adams." *The Missourian*, June 24, 1820.

[3]Albert Gallatin Boone (1806–84), grandson of Daniel Boone, would have been about nineteen years old when he traveled with Dr. Willard in 1825. A. G. Boone was born in Greensburg, Kentucky, and moved with the Boone clan to Saint Charles County, Missouri. At age seventeen he joined the second Ashley-Henry trapping party out of Saint Louis traveling to the Upper Missouri. He worked for a while at the Fort Osage trading post in western Missouri mastering the Osage language and learning several other native tongues. He later served as deputy county clerk of Saint Charles County before moving to Callaway County, where he worked in his brother-in-law's tobacco business. In 1838 he established his own trading business in Westport. Charles Clark, http://kansasboguslegislature.org/mo/boone_a_g.html (accessed August 10, 2011).

[4]The Chariton River is 218 miles long and has been called Missouri's Grand Divide, as the streams east of it flow to the Mississippi River and the streams west flow into the Missouri River. Several origins of the name Chariton have been suggested. The most plausible suggestion connects the name of the river with Joseph Chorette, a French fur trader of Saint Louis. Trudeau, in his *Journal* of 1795, mentions that Chorette accompanied him on his expedition up the Missouri River and drowned on July 10 of that year while swimming in the river. The family name has the variants Choret, Care, and Carrette in old documents. "Origins of Missouri Counties," http://www.sos.mo.gov/archives/history/counties.asp (accessed August 20, 2011).

fearing I might need for something made it available this occasion. I saw that night was at my heels & the wilderness seemed unbroken & hense expedition alone could relieve me from present dilema. I took my rope & tied one to my riding horses bridle & thru uncoiling my rope slung it a cross the stream, lodging the end upon the other bank, and stripping my horses of everything carried it over on my back a cross a tree which spanned the river, & when all was over, caught the end of my rope & pulled my horse into the stream the other followed swimming over to my embrace I soon had them saddled & on my way. I got to Franklin after dark having rode through alternate showers all day.

Put up with Captain Means with who I was some acquainted but more particularly with his daughter Eliza[5] who had spent the previous winter at St. Charles & with whom I had passed several convivial evenings.

Finding me on my way to Mexico, they proposed assisting me to my outfit. The Negroes were set to baking crackers for my journey which took them nearly all night.

In the morning early Mr. Marble & Mr. [Mc]Knight arrived they having chased me all the way from St. Charles. They were also destined for Mexico & needed the same outfit as myself & hense the poor Negroes had no respite, but forced to continue their cracker trade.

At this place I met with an old acquaintance by the name of Storrs a grocer. He professed to know what all we wanted. I told him to procure everything necessary, which he did with great clarraty. He went to the trimmers, & ordered for us six canteens for water, a pair of hobbles for each horse, Tea, Sugar, salt & etc. etc. etc.

The 2nd batch of crackers having been baked, & everything in readiness, we were on our way, much relieved of my former loneliness. We arrived at Lexington[6] on the eve of the 13th where we tarried for one

---

[5]Eliza Ann Alexander Means (1800–?), ancestry.com, accessed June 7, 2013.

[6]From the early 1820s until the Civil War, Lexington, located in western Missouri, was involved in almost every aspect of the Santa Fe trade. Lexington's first settler was probably Gillad Rupe, who came to the area around 1815 from Boonville, where he had operated a ferry. He may have started a ferry at the mouth of "Rupe's branch" on the Missouri, but by 1819 Captain William Jack was known to be operating the ferry. "Jack's Ferry Road" was the connection between the river and the early settlement centered about two miles to the east. Lexington was platted in 1822 in the area later known as "Old Town" and became the county seat in 1823 with a log courthouse in a public square. Direct expeditions from the Lexington area started as early as 1822 when Strother Renick, whose family had settled seven miles west at Wellington, *(continued)*

day for Marble & [McK]night to lay in their goods. The next day we left the settlement & struck out into the wilderness & travelled 30 miles where we overtook the main company.[7] Here I spread my tent for the 1st time.

The next morning was pleasant, & everything looked novel & interesting. Among the company I found several with whom I had been partially acquainted, & who greeted me with hearty welcome. After breakfast, the packers concluded that it would be expedient to sepparate ourselves from the main company & go forward believing we could out travel the wagons.

We accordingly took our leave & proceeded to the Blue Springs[8] some ten miles distant, and then halted to organize our company by choosing R. M. Morris for our Captain & J. Fultcher, as Lieutenant also Sargeants of the guards. Being now organized we set forth taking our course, by the compass, ranging as we found it necessary to avoid untenible grounds & difficult streams. I have now before me a daily entry of that tour but I shall only notice the most interesting incidents without following in detail the diary in which I was particular in noting the precise time of starting and stopping, thus computing the hours of travel, which I multiplied by three in order that I might compute the whole distance.[9] After getting into what is now called Kansas, we encountered some 20 Sack Indians who being on horseback accompanied us several miles.

---

was hired by a General McRea to "take a small stock of goods on pack mules over the trackless prairie to Mexico." Renick was only nineteen and afterward made several similar trips by himself. He is said to have specialized in trading for mules. For trail historians, the first really significant business in Lexington was the store and warehouse built by John Aull, who came from Delaware in 1822. He was followed by his brothers Robert and James Aull in 1825. "Lexington, Missouri and the Santa Fe Trail," http://www.santafetrailresearch.com/research/lexington-mo.html (accessed August 23, 2011).

[7]Willard would rendezvous with the company at Fort Osage, Missouri.

[8]During the earliest period of the Santa Fe Trail (1821–27), one of the routes left Fort Osage and went south following the road that connected Fort Osage to Harmony Mission. On this route the Blue Springs Campground was an important rendezvous point. Other traders came to Blue Springs directly from Lexington, and from Cooper, Saline and Howard Counties in Missouri. Simmons and Jackson, *Following the Santa Fe Trail*, 45–46.

[9]The Rowland Willard pocket diary of Dr. Willard's western journey to New Mexico and Mexico (1825–27) is part of the Yale Collection of Western Americana at the Beinecke Rare Book and Manuscript Library, Rowland Willard and Elizabeth S. Willard Papers, WA MSS S-2512. All references to the pocket diary and autobiography are to this source.

They appeared quite Civil, & seemed to have no other business than to trade horses with us & sell some skins & moccasins. Mr. Cave swapped horses with them, he having one addicted to throwing his rider but the young Indian not being aware of his trick, put spur to him, when he soon found himself sprawling in the grass. He jumped up with apparent surprise, giving a lusty whoop as he saw his treacherous steed sailing arround until it reached the company again. The company halted a little while some assisted in catching his pony.

Our general course was southwest until we reached the Arkansas River. Our game at first consisted of deer & antelope, droves of elk were often seen, but quite shy, thus we could not get a shot at them. When we came to what we then termed the little Arkansas (a tributary of the main Arkansas) we found fresh signs of Buffalo. Several hunters went forward to take them by stealth, & brought into camp an abundance of beef. The next day we met the herd whose members could not be computed. I estimated the numbers seen that day to 100,000. It might be more & it might be less. The country seemed covered as far as vision could reach with buffalo. The great park of nature seemed boundless & altho filled mostly with buffalo, yet the Elk, Deer, Antelope, Wolf & Fox were occasionally seen among them.

At the Blue Springs we found in waiting 4 men whose names were Stone,[10] Glass, March[11] & Andrews,[12] who desired to accompany us for the purpose of hunting & trapping on the head water of the Rio [Bravo] del Norte.

When we came up to them, they presented us with plenty of venison which they had killed, while laying there awaiting our arrival. It appeared that they had started with each a mule & an outfit of traps but in crossing a bad stream, lost three of their mules & many of their traps. And having but one mule left their remaining traps &

---

[10]Solomon Stone was a partner with Alexander Branch in several fur-trapping expeditions. Stone applied for Mexican citizenship in November of 1826 through Governor Antonio Narbona. Weber, *Taos Trappers*, 122, 176.

[11]In the pocket diary entries for July 10 and 12, 1825, Dr. Willard refers to Stephen Marsh. Marsh is ordered by Major Henry to accompany Hugh Glass on an expedition to Fort Atkinson. Manfred, *Lord Grizzly*, 222–23.

[12]In Dr. Willard's pocket diary he refers to a John Andrews in his entry dated September 16, 1825.

baggage proved a load for it, & they obliged to walk. These men had been several trips among the mountains for Beaver. But it mattered little whether they got much or little, for when arriving to the settlement, would debauch until all was spent, & then off again, at least such I was told was the case with Stone, & Glass, the former a middle aged man, but Glass was quite advanced in life probably 75. He was by birth a Highland Scotch man, & still retained the kilts & cap of his native country. In his selection of Messrs, seemed rather inclined to fraternise with Mr. Rennisons[13] mess, & the one I belonged to & hense his game, which he killed almost daily was mostly brought to our messes he being considered *our* hunter. On one occasion he went out just prior to coming to the Buffalo, & chanced to meet with an Indian horse, which he found had been ridden. He managed to make a bridle of bark, and succeeded in catching him, & who should come riding up at night but father Glass delighted with his game.

In this place it may be well to record briefly, a portion of the old man's history as related to me by himself. It seems that during a prior excursion among the mountains with these same comrads, & while trapping for beavers, I think that the four above mentioned had singled themselves from the main company, & were trapping on their own "hook." He said that he was on camp duty one morning while the rest were out to examine their traps. And as he was busy in cooking about the fire, there suddenly came upon him a large white Bear[14] who

---

[13] The *Missouri Intelligencer* published the following on June 4, 1825: "Among the packers who are in advance are Messrs. Morris and Rennison, of Howlud, Mr. Barnes of Boon, Dr. Willard, of St. Charles and two gentlemen from Natchez." "Santa Fe Adventurers," *Missouri Intelligencer*, June 4, 1825. A list of trail traders who paid 15 percent importation duty and 3 percent excise tax at the Santa Fe customhouse indicated that on July 8, 1825, a John Remison [Rennison] from Franklin (Howard County, Missouri) presented an original trade invoice dated April 30, 1825. Weber, *Extranjeros*, 17.

[14] The reference to the white bear is a grizzly bear that attacked Hugh Glass in 1823 when he was employed by Maj. Henry as a trapper at Grand River, South Dakota. A newspaper article published on Hugh Glass states, "The rifle of Hugh Glass being esteemed as among the most unerring, he was on one occasion detached for supplies. He was a short distance in advance of the party, and forcing his way through a thicket, when a white bear that had imbedded herself in the sand, arose, within three yards of him, and before he could 'set his triggers,' or turn to retreat, he was seized by the throat, and raised from the ground. Casing him again upon the earth, his grim adversary tore out a mouthful of a cannibal food which had excited her appetite, and retired to submit the sample to her yearling cubs, which were near at hand. The sufferer now made an effort to escape, but the bear immediately returned with a reinforcement,

unceremoniously laid hold of him and threw him down, & immediately commenced his work of destruction. In this disastrous condition, the old man lay with the monster mounted upon him when Mr. Stone chanced to return from his traps with rifle in hand, & seeing the awful predicament of his comrad, leveled his piece & to his great satisfaction the monster fell dead upon his victim.

I examined the old man who stripped off his clothes & showed me the large chasms upon right arm & shoulder blade the crest of which was wanting, also the upper portions of the right thigh. The history he gave of the matter was well attested, both by Stone & by ocular proof.

At this time the Indians became hostile in their aspect & it was thought best to get the general Co together, & hold a consultation, in reference not only to Glass, but to themselves also. It was decided that the company should leave that district, and make their way towards the upper settlement of Missouri, or beyond the range of that tribe.

This being decided upon it was imposible to take the tortured old man with them, & what must be done with him. He was yet alive, & to leave him alone to other disasters, would be a mark of great inhumanity and it was therefore agreed that each man on arriving to St. Louis with their furs, should pay to any two men who should consent to stay with him until he should die ten dollars. This offer was accepted by two young men[15] & the rest took this departure. They staid with him 4 days & left, following the trail of the company until they overtook it, & reported that the old man had died before they left. Some of this company either went or wrote to St Louis & stated the facts of Glass's death & it was published I think in the Missouri Republican[16]

---

and seized him again at the shoulder; she also lacerated his left arm very much, and inflicted a severe wound on the back of his head. In the second attack, the cubs were prevented from participating by one of the party, who had rushed forward to the relief of his comrade. One of the cubs, however, forced the new comer to retreat into the river, where, standing to the middle in water, he gave his foe a mortal shot. Meantime the main body of trappers having arrived, advanced to the relief of Glass and delivered seven or eight shots with such unerring aim as to terminate hostilities, by dispatching the bear as she stood over her victim. Glass was thus snatched from the grasp of the ferocious animal, yet his condition was far from being enviable." "The Missouri Trapper," *Missouri Intelligencer*, June 18, 1825.

[15] The two young men who accepted the award offered by Maj. Henry were John Fitzgerald and James Bridger. Lamar, *New Encyclopedia*, 431–32.

[16] In 1821 the name of this Saint Louis newspaper, the first newspaper west of the Mississippi, was changed from *Missouri Gazette* to *Missouri Republican*. The founder was Joseph Charless.

that old Mr. Glass had been eaten up by a White Bear. But it was not exactly so, Glass was yet alive, & I was able to identify him myself.

It seems from what he told me, that about the time the young men left, his wounds began to sepparate as the inflammation gave way, followed by a healing action. The weather was warm, & their provisions being meat only, soon spoiled, & hense starvation seemed to stare the old man in the face; but fortunately he was left near a spring of water, to which he could crawl upon his hands & knees. In a few days more, came to the conclusion to work his way upon the trail of the company, and gleaning as he went such roots as he could masticate for food, and I think he had not gone far, before he could bear his weight upon his legs and finally succeeded in overtaking the company which had commence[d] trapping again.

The surprise of the company may be imagined on seeing him appear among them, as well as the consternation of the two young men left with him to stay with him until he should die.

But the old man lived to go once more, & one only without a return. He said to me "I am old, but I thought I would go out once more Doctor, but I think it will be my last," & sure enough it was. When I entered the village of Taos the old man met me with enthusiasm & tried to bear me on his shoulders saying that I had saved his life on the way, during a turn of the colic. He had got in a few hours before me & had met with his old idol that induced you to inebriation. To finish up his biography I will here remark that he went out with a company of mostly French men, to hunt on the waters of the Colorado he with several others, fell a victim to his credulity having put confidence in a party of Indians who fell upon them in the night with clubs & he lies on the eastern side of the Pacific instead of the eastern side of the Atlantic his native land.

But to return, on the 1st of June [1825] we came to a prairie Dog town, which was the first I had seen, and which to me was rather interesting, exhibiting as they did a kind of domestic polity. Their domiciliary arrangements being vicinal, or gregarious, insomuch that we termed them "dog towns" when we passed through their communities. Our approach was always announced by the abundant barking of their vigilant sentinels, who sat perched upon the little mounds at the mouths of their subterranian dwellings. Their clamorous barking resembling that of the domestic foxes, tho they offered no resistance or challenge, but retired within their holes in confident safety. They were clumsily built, rather bull headed of short hair reddish colour, & little less in size than the Spanish lapdog & were it not for their barking might have been domesticated Feline instead of Canine; one of which species I think they will belong to.

We now pursued our way up the Arkansas River, occasionally cutting off its larger bends but confined to its waters daily. As we encamped on the 3rd came upon two buffalo laying burried near the waters edge. I proposed to the boys that we would make an effort to extricate them from their present dilemma by putting a rope around their horns & dragging them from their confinement. They agreed in my proposition but the poor animals were so far spent that self assistance was no longer available, and they had quietly to succumb to their fate.

About this time the distant sand hills[17] made their singular appearance, & to one unaccustomed to their illusive mirage,[18] the effect upon the senses was quite peculiar.

In this instance, the appearance was that of flames of fire resembling a burning prairie. These apparent flames would mount per saltum[19] to the hight of fifteen or twenty feet, exhibiting the brilliant agitation peculiar to prairie fires driven with strong winds. This fiery aspect finally changed into an apparent sheet of water which for some time challenged my credibility which was almost irresistible until I found the approaching lake to recede before us. In accounting for this strange phenomenon I apprehend that the impinging surface casting an unequal refraction from the numerous repeling surfaces of the sand, into the

---

[17]These sand hills could be Plum Buttes, three enormous sand mounds that were well known as trail landmarks but are greatly diminished today. They were once located between Lyons and Great Bend, in western Rice County, Kansas. Franzwa, *Maps*, 80–81.

[18]Numerous travelers, including Albert Pike, Josiah Gregg, Lewis H. Garrard, Marion Russell, and soldiers stationed at military forts, described mirages on the Santa Fe Trail. Morgan, "Mirages on the Santa Fe Trail," 8–11.

[19]*Per saltum:* "At a leap; without passing through intermediate stages or steps," or in this context "quickly changing." http://m.wordnik.com/words/per%20saltum (accessed September 3, 2011).

stratum of atmosphere contiguous to the earth producing effects similar to that of descending rain drops between us & the sun, which gives the beautiful colours of the rainbows. These optical illusions I have met with but three or four times in my travels, and seem to occur at a certain altitude of the sun and yet, it would seem that nothing less than a complication of phenomena, will produce the illusive effect.

The refraction obliquity of the sun rays cannot alone claim the phenomenon else it would appear daily & universally at such an altitude of the sun, and such an obliquity of the refracted rays.

About this place our bread gave out having lasted some fifteen days, & we were now reduced to less than a Cape Cod variety,[20] even to a unite,[21] meat being our only article of subsistence, but if any meat will relish & maintain its applicancy to the wants of nature it is the tender buffalo beef. We had now met the great herd or drove as they were feeding northwardly, & we travelling southwesterly their numbers became so dense, that it became necessary to keep out riders to their course & keep our caravan clear of them; but before we finally apprehended our danger, a considerable accident occurred. The great mass of buffalo had become disturbed, or agitated, & an almost simultaneous rush in the same direction. As they approached so near us & paid but little attention to us until they came quite near us, I proposed to Mr. Marble to lead my riding horse that I might move forward & try my luck in killing one. In attempting to shoot missed fire, I then took out my knife to pick the flint, in this act, the buffalo coming suddenly

---

[20]"A hard, small bread or roll among the Quakers. It was usually served at breakfast or at afternoon tea. In flavor, the traditional Quaker rusks were faintly sweet; in color, they were deep yellow (from the eggs) with dark brown tops. In the country, they were usually eaten fresh, although technically a true rusk should be dry and brittle because it is dried out in a slack oven. At one time, rusks were a fairly widespread feature of urban Anglo-American cookery, at least on the East Coast [Cape Cod]. They were introduced from England, where they were popularly served as shipboard fare, as dried rusks should be laid down in tins or stored for long periods of time. The name, however, is of foreign origin and may be derived from the Spanish or Portuguese *rosca*, a twist or roll of bread. Such small breads often served as part of the traveling fare for Spanish or Portuguese sailors." William Woys Weaver, *A Quaker Woman's Cookbook: The Domestic Cookery of Elizabeth Ellicott Lea* (Mechanicsburg, Penn.: Stackpole Books, 2004), 341; Lynn Olver, "The Food Timeline: Cookies, Crackers, and Biscuits," http://www.foodtimeline.org/foodcookies.html (accessed August 26, 2011).

[21]*unite:* Willard's meaning is unclear.

upon me, a few turned & ran between me & the company which had approached pretty near me. In their affrighted bound, some six horses travelling loose took fright and sprang in with them and went off at full speed. The owners were all on horseback save one man, & instantly gave chase & after a while succeeded in separating them from the heard & got them back their former allegiance. But our Lieutenant Mr. Fulcher like myself was forward experimenting with his rifle. And when his horses were recognized by him among the buffalo, he could but stand to regret his delinquency in not attending to his own interest. No one offered him a horse at the moment & the three horses belonging to him were directly commingled with the heard of buffalo, together with all he had except the clothes on his back. His goods cost him $300 for which he had mortgaged his farm in Missouri.

I felt rather implicated as being accessory to the accident having turned the course of the buffalo but it was an incidence I could not forsee nor was I ever censured by the company to my knowledge, but feeling as I did for the unfortunate man I proposed to the Captain that we should encamp immediately that search might be made for the lost horses. He accordingly called a halt & after taking a refreshment, myself & another volunteered to follow them some 6 or 8 miles. We returned without them. In the evening seven of us volunteered to go again hoping we might chance to come upon them, we took around the bend of the river & continued our course until dark when we hobbled horses & lay down. At midnight I was told by the man on guard that my mare had got footloose and had ran off from the gang taking with her another horse belonging to lawyer Cave. The mare having been loaned me by Mr. Marble (my own being tired) I felt the more anxious to recover her, & proposed to Mr. Cave that we sally forth immediately, but the night being somewhat dark, succeed to hesitate, & it was not until I started alone that he made up his mind to accompany me.

We steared in the direction of the main camp as near as we could apprehend the course & travelled about an hour when I thought I heard a voice floating upon the air & immediately stoped & listened. The faint vibration was again recognized & we found it a human voice.

I said to Mr. C.[ave] that it was probably the horses had returned &
that we would return to the camp we had left & thereupon made our
way back again. As we neared them daylight begun to brake, & in
coming to them, found shure enough, our horses were there before us.

After masticating a little buffalo beef we started again & persued our
course separating from each other, and travelling until the afternoon
without seing any sign of horses, when I turned towards camp arriving
a little before night. The men all arrived about the same time without
success. Next morning the company concluded to pursue our journey,
sending out several men in hopes yet to find the horses, agreeing to
meet up the river, at our place of encampment.

The men all came in at night with the exception of Andrews.

By this time Mr. Fultcher became rather discouraged, & began to
question the propriety of pursuing his journey, saying that he had a
farm & family at home, and by returning could make his time good
on his farm.

We felt that it would be presumptious to think of returning alone,
and accordingly the Company proposed to pay him wages while
detained in Mexico for the hearding [of] their horses, and I also drew
up a subscription for him, to which was subscribed 145.00 to remunerate in some measure his loss.

Hitherto my two messmates Marble & Knight had been antagonis-
tich in their feelings, & wholly taciturn consequent to Marble having claimed the best horse as being a purchase of his own whereas
Knight claimed it to be a company purchase. This personal association
had become grossly obnoxious & their odium increased daily. Their
Goods having been purchased together could not be easily divided,
nevertheless a division was insisted upon, & the parties decided that
I should make it. The packs were therefore unbound, & each piece
of goods unfolded, while I gave each an end which being brought
together. I found the middle & taring in two gave each his half &
thus everything was divided with scrupulous equality & each made
again his own bundle.

Having divided goods, it was insisted that the mess should be divided
also. And it was propounded which I would retain as mess mate.

Having no special prefference I would not decide. Marble seemed quite tenacious of his preference to remain. Knight went to himself & joined no other mess on the way. As my Mess had so long been in a state of anarchy & even mutiny I felt relieved when their interests were surrendered.

The next day we arrived at Pawney Creek[22] which we found so deep, that it could not be forded, with safety, to our goods. A raft was therefore constructed of old limbs &c gathered on the shore, upon which the goods were crossed with safety, & the mules & horses made to swim.

That night we shot guns as a guide to Andrews who had not yet arrived.

Mr. Fultcher had now become satisfied, that his duties required him to return to his family. His mind having been, better to try it, many of the company concluded to make him post boy, & accordingly wrote back to their friends.

A horse was furnished him by one of his neighbours & provisions was abundant on the way made necessary by his rifle. Breakfast being over, he commenced the parting ceremony with tears in his eyes, conscious of the dangers that might lurk in the way. But he was a man of considerable fortitude & perseverance & he commenced retracing his steps with hope of being once more in the bosom of his family. While plodding his way upon the prairie adjoining the river on I think & the 3rd day of his return, he fortunately stumbled upon his best packs which had been thrown by the animals & was uninjured. This unexpected good fortune changed his course again, & he was resolved to see Mexico provided nothing should thwart his purpose. He slung his packs upon his horse, & hurried back to the Pawney Creek determined to await there the arrival of the waggons. And lest they might pass it while he should be out in pursuit of game, wrote advertisements which he put up at several places on the river or creek when he thought they might chance to cross. I think that in about a week the waggons arrived found him in waiting. He accompanied

---

[22]Pawnee Creek, Pawnee Fork, and Pawnee River are all the same. It was located on the Wet Route, which was used by Santa Fe Trail travelers before the 1830s, near the location of present-day Larned, Kansas. Simmons and Jackson, *Following the Santa Fe Trail*, 120–26.

them until he came to the Spanish pass to Taos when he struck off by himself, & crossed the mountains alone.

When he arrived [in Taos] I assisted him in passing his goods through the Custom House with but little duty, & he was off directly among the inhabitants unaided by an interpreter, when he disposed of his little sacks for money & mules & stood in readiness for a home journey long before the rest of the company.

But to return. On the eleventh we passed two vaults of some 8 or 10 feet diameter, where a company had cashed their goods some 18 ms. ago & who having started late in the fall became rather bound at this place having encountered a great snowstorm falling to the depth of three to four feet & utterly precluding their further progress. It so happened that their encampment was in an isolated grove of cotton wood which supplied them with fuel for the winter & material for a hut. Three mules browsed for a while upon the brush of the grove but was insufficient to their maintenance & the depth of the snow precluded access to the grass & consequently they all perished before spring. As the snow melted away they found it necessary to make some shift to get to the settlement, and their plan was to bury their goods in the cashes or excavations before mentioned. Covering them over sufficiently as to elude the suspicions of the savage tribes, which might pass that way. They laid poles over, then brush, & lastly the earth excavated rounding it off nicely, & then the better to conceal their work of art, killed two Buffalo & draged their carcases over the mounds, that the wolves might in their rapine efface the diggings & deceive the passing redmen.

I would here observe that their own means of support consisted of buffalo obtained with some difficulty as they were scarce & could only be reached upon Snow Shoes. But in this way they subsisted until Spring when they all walked into Taos where they obtained more mules, which they returned with & found their concealed goods in a state of perfect safety.

On the 12th the hunters shot four buffalo which supplied us abundantly. I thought much upon domestic associations & comforts, of which I was then deprived, but I endeavoured to act the philosopher, hoping to reach sivilization again in about twenty days. We were the

more tried having become drenched though successive showers, &
thereby greatly incommoded. But the genial Sun soon dissipated the
atmospheric clouds & the mutual gloom gave way also.

On the 14th we stopped to refresh & having occasion to shave,
opened my trunk which I found taking damage in consequence of my
acid bottle leaking the stopple having got loose. In order to secure it,
the Captain delayed a little which enabled our last man Andrews to
get within sight of us & immediately discharged his rifle to hail our
attention. Being on the river bottom, we could see a long distance, &
hearing the report of a gun our attention was called that way, & as I
looked down the river I could see a man running toward us with all his
might I said, "there comes Andrews," and sure enough a few minutes
brought him to our recognition. His arrival was hailed with hearty
means & we all stood anxious to learn of his adventurous absence. In
a few words he informed us that on the first day of his horse excursion, he was espied by a party of Indians who made him prisoner & as
they were travelling downstream, daily sundered us farther & farther.
Moreover they crossed the river & after travelling two or three days
he stole from them in the dead of night while all lay asleep.

He found with them a coat lost by our company which together with
an elegant buffalo robe which he purloined, made his way up the river
as fast as possible. Being on the south side of the [Arkansas] river he
concluded to cross over in order to get upon our trail & how to get
over with his plunder, he could not devise. His rifle & ammunition
was indispensible as his subsistence depended on them, & to swim
with them all he found was impracticable & hense was compelled to
throw away his coat & robe and with the aid of a dry limb which he
placed under his breast he navigated the river with his rifle tied upon
his back. After getting again upon the north side, he could find our
encampments at night & towards the last the fires were still burning.
This encouraged him to make rapid strides until he overtook us which
was after being absent from us eight days. He said the Indians showed
no signs of evil toward him, but treated him kindly.

We tarried on the 15th & 16th to lay in our meat for the rest of the
journey. Several hunters went out a mile or two distance from camp,

while I accompanied them to witness the game of taking such brutes without risk of life or limb & with but little comparative exercise or skill. We had not gone far before we discovered six or eight fine bulls by themselves, the country being entirely clear of bushes, or any other ambuscade as soon as we came in sight of them we were obliged to disguise ourselves & approach them as quadrupeds instead of bipeds, hense upon all fours. This was an unpleasant mode of travel, but our success depended on the adroitness of our address, using the utmost caution to conceal our species. Any quadruped could be tollerated tho ever so monstrous, but an erect posture, & the face of men strikes dread upon the whole brute creation.

We continued our awkward gambol until we got within shooting distance. Mr. Cave & myself were scouting latterally, while the better hunters were approaching them directly, & served as fuglemen[23] for us. When they placed the hat for resting the rifle upon it, I did likewise & as soon as they fired I followed suit. At the crack of the rifle, one of the buffalo started a little walk a kind of flirt but did not offer to run nor did the rest scare. The hunter lay & loaded again, & by that time the wounded one began to cough & at length lay down. We saw that he was quite safe. The second one was now selected, & when a side proposition was had, the fatal bull frustrated his lungs, & he too soon laid down while we arose to our feet & the rest ran off.

We now commenced skinning with caution as the hides were to serve us as boats in which to ferry the river. After removing the hide we commenced flaying the muscles & packing our horses, my own being quite docile. I had got some 100 pounds laid upon her, but happening to turn her head, she discovered the gory load & sprang to get away from it, when the meat flew right & left she taking a circuitous rout gradually came to us again when I caught her.

The meat was then laid upon the more gentle burden bearers, & I had the pleasure of riding into camp instead of leading.

We then flayed the meat, & hung it upon lines stretched for the purpose, where it became dry the next day & fit for packing. While

---

[23]Guides.

our "jerk" was drying we made two skin boats by sewing up the bull hides, then tying four sticks at the corners commenced lacing up the edge of the hide, converting it into tub form. With these two tub boats we crossed all the goods with perfect safety. Two mule loads were put into the tub & then Mr. Rennison & myself & got in on top & were floated across by a man on each side, fording most the way, but swimming the channel. The next morning we started again; tho I would remark before passing, that Andrews in attempting to cross the river on his mule got tangled in some brush & to save his life was obliged to throw away his rifle, being now reduced to a few traps & a little ammunition, but such men are just as happy without as with possessions.

We now followed up on the south side of the river, seeing occasionally droves of wild horses, but could not approach them. The hunters killed 5 or 6 buffalo, furnishing us with an abundance of fresh meat.

We now concluded to leave the Arkansas River crossing[24] through the sand hills to the SimiRone river, a distance of some 45 miles ~~distance~~. In this crossing, water is seldom found altho we chanced to meet with a small pond it having recently rained. It was for this part of the road that we needed our canteens, & on leaving the river every man was careful to fill all the vessels that would hold water, & we tied up a large sack of it in an oil cloth, but the weather being quite warm, rendered it unpalatable & could not be drank. I could but notice the increase of thirst when reduced to a meat competency.

We encamped by this little pond regarding ourselves fortunate in having encountered it. At this encampment I had fresh meat laying near my head, which was taken before morning as I supposed by the wolves made bold by hunger. This transit from river to river, was often attended with peril, owning to the SimiRone's being a venial stream supplied from the snows of the mountains & made larger or shorter according to circumstances.

---

[24]This would be the Upper Crossing of the Arkansas River before traveling south along the Cimarron Route. It begins south of present-day Lakin, Kansas, leading first to Chocteau's Island and following the drainage of Bear Creek in western Kansas. Simmons and Jackson, *Following the Santa Fe Trail*, 136, 172.

Mr. Rennison informed me that the year before he had well nigh perished. The river being dry was passed over supposed to be nothing more than a ravine. The Company urging forward in expectation of meeting the river was at length compeled to conclude they had passed it, & to return back to the Arkansas before they could relieve their thirst.

Several had become so despondent that they lay down in the prairie, & would have perished, but for a few more persevering who reached the river & after slaking their thirst, returned with water to resuscitate the famished ones. The same difficulty occured the next year after I passed through, as related to me by Mr. Scott who stopped with me some months at Chihuahua where he followed the silversmith trade. He described their anxiety as amounting to a state of desperation becoming reckless of everything but self preservation. One of his mules laden with silversmith tools strayed off & was lost, so utterly worthless was everything but water for which they were famishing. This pass was the most formidable obstruction on the way although the Indians were quite hostile for several years after I passed through.

On the 21st I had the mortification to lose one of my pistols my mare having taken fright at the wolf skin fastened to the saddle as it flitted in the wind. The pistol was thrown from the holster as she ran, they were a favorite brace & I exceedingly disliked to part with it. Having been delayed in starting made her the more uneasy to overtake the company which she soon caught up with & was caught & retained until my arrival with the other which was packed. My old friend Rennison seeing my difficulty, who together with McKnight volunteered their assistance to find it. We were able occasionally to discover, our trace in the grass & which we followed a little sepperated from each other until we at length came upon it. Further Rennison first discovered it, when he cried out "I have found it" as much alerted as if he had found a fortune. We now hurried on feeling ourselves fully compensated for our pains but it was some hours before we overtook the company.

The Simi Rone we found without current although the holes were filled with water into which the buffalo were frequently plunging for water keeping it constantly, turbid & filthy. We could not drink it in that state but with a spade would dig a hole a little one side into which the water would distill, but it was more like barnyard than like river water.

We did not travel many days on this river, before we came to springs, the country becoming a little more broken with here & there a knob or rocky hillock skirted with cedar.

Near this part of the rout we espied at a distance a caravan moving northward which was thought by some to be Indians but proved to be a company of Americans & Spaniards on their way to Missouri. Don [Manuel] Escudero[25] a somewhat prominent citizen of Chihuahua being among them & whose family I afterwards became acquainted with. On the 25th we passed two prominent isolated knobs standing wholly separate & so nearly contiguous as that they were denominated "Rabbit Ears" and regarded as way marks to the traders then, but now probably not so heeded, as a plain beaten road now obtains. We also

---

[25]Governor Baca "commissioned a special envoy to negotiate with American authorities for its protection from the Indians of the intermediate plains. This envoy was Manual Simón Escudero, a member of the Chihuahua legislature. Accompanying a Missouri caravan returning from Santa Fé, Escudero obtained a favorable recommendation from the United States Indian agent at St. Louis and laid the New Mexican proposals before the Mexican minister at Washington. They were the first known Mexican merchants to trade with the United States by way of the Santa Fe Trail." Moorhead, *New Mexico's Royal Road*, 66. Escudero traveled in the company of American trader Meredith Miles Marmaduke, the future governor of Missouri; and two Mexican merchants, Ramon Garcia from Chihuahua and Rumualdo Garcia from Sonora and their servants. The pack train consisted of six hundred horses and mules. "When the caravan reached the United States, a St. Louis newspaper reported that it contained seventeen Americans and twenty-three Mexicans, the latter from El Paso, Chihuahua and Sonora. Among the Mexicans, the newspaper reported, in a clear reference to Escudero, was 'a gentleman of wealth and distinction in his own country, a member of the Mexican Congress [the paper mistook the Chihuahua Congress for the national Congress], but whose name we cannot undertake to write from the Pronunciation we have heard of it.'" Weber, "Señor Escudero Goes to Washington," 425. A year later, according to the *Missouri Intelligencer*, "Six or seven new and substantial built waggons arrived in this place on Tuesday last, heavily laden with merchandise, on their way to New Mexico, owned exclusively, we believe, by Mr. Escudero, a native of that country, and who accompanies his valuable adventure. This gentleman has expended a very large sum in the purchase of goods, waggons and equipment. This may be considered as a new era in the commerce between Mexico and his country, and it is probable the example of Mr. E will be followed by others of his rich countrymen, who will bring hither large portions of their surplus wealth, for the same purpose." *Missouri Intelligencer*, June 9, 1826, 3. Between 1821 and 1838 Escudero was the only "Hispano who travelled east to purchase manufactures directly in the United States." Boyle, *Los Capitalistas*, 60–61.

passed another knob quite isolated, we climbed up to the summit &
found evident signs of usual defense & no doubt the work of savage
tribes.

We now began to descry the rock, mountains at a great distance.
Mr. Storrs the hunter remarked that their fartherest promontory could
not be less than one hundred miles distant. They approach luminous
on their snow capped summits denoting their great altitude.

We now came to a creek which we supposed to be a tributary of the
Red River. We met with alternate showers during a day and night,
greatly incommoding us. As we were confined to buffalo manure for
fuel, it was quite difficult to make fire & at one time was done at the
expense of old shirts, & a quantity of tallow.

Our clothes & blankets had become saturated during the day, & not
being able to make a fire were obliged to lay down cold & wet. After
getting a little warm, we were aroused by the water running under
us, obliged to move our moorings to higher ground. Having got quiet
again the guard reported that a part of the horses were missing & some
seemed confident that Indians were about. I ascertained that my own
horses were safe and then reloaded my rifle & pistols preparatory to
any exigency that might arise. Much consternation was manifested
among such as missed their animals, & trouble was fully accredited,
but Mr. Rennison concluded to make search & walking down the
creek a short distance discovered the lost herd. It appeared that the
first guard went on duty late, and a portion of the animals had got
one side, & undiscovered in the fore part of the night.

On the 1st day of July we began in the afternoon to ascend the
mountains. It had been quite sultry during the day, but as we began to
ascend a pleasant a breeze sprang up, while the aspect of water seemed
constantly to change. We encamped on the side of the mountain upon
the Spanish trail. Here we lay by a beautiful cold spring with wood
& grass plenty around us. The snow had mostly melted except in low
places into which it had been drifted.

The next day we got within 12 miles of Taos & encamped. We were
proceeded by a few who by forced march had conveyed intelligence of
our approach, and the *Alcalde* suspicious of our smuggling came out

in the morning with 10 or dozen to meet us. They brought with them *Tortillas* & caso [*queso*] (pancakes & cheese).

All goods were taken into custody except my own & placed under guard until next day.

The Alcade learning that I was a physician said I might pass on to town which soon hove in sight. He soon followed me & commenced conversation in Spanish, while I replied negatively in French "Non Tompa." He conducted me to his house where the family gather around me as if I had been a nondescript. I was seated on the banca [*banco*, e.g., bench] composed of wool mattresses (*colchóns*) rolled up matting, and soft convenient seat making across the end of the parlour (*sala*). The old man made several attempts to converse with me, but not a word did I comprehend. The Indian dialect would have been quite as intelligible, & hense to every question I gracefully nodded "non tompe" a Monsieur.

We had not sat long however, before a domestic Indian girl approached, and placing a little bench (*banca*) before us spreading over it a white cloth. She then came with two earthen plates of stewed flesh-coloured beans and a few pancakes made of corn ground by hand & not an implement of any kind to eat with. How I was to succeed I could not yet descipher but thought to myself that if he could manage to eat them, I could follow suit in some sort. After a short ceremony of Catholic grace he proceeded to the task of tearing a pancake in two and doubling the half scooped fearlessly into his plate of beans, & the mystery was solved. I found the thing practicable to a hungry man not bad to take.

After dinner I went out into the village & soon met with a Frenchman by the name of Antoine Rubideaux[26] who learning I had stopped with the *Alcade*, advised me to go a mile into the country & board with him, as the old man did not maintain the best of character. I accordingly accompanied him to the house of Don Pablo Lucero a worthy old farmer & by the by a good kind of a man. He charged me twelve dollars per month for board & treated me with kindness.

---

[26]Antoine Robidoux (1794–1860), one of six brothers born in Florissant, Missouri. He was part of the first Atkinson-Long expedition of 1818–19, which reached the site of Council Bluffs, Iowa. In 1822–23 he made his first trip to Santa Fe.

It was soon rumored that I was a physician, & calls for medical aid were prompt & continuous. I usually visited town every day, & was greatly amused in witnessing the manners & customs of a simi savage people, the most of whom had never passed the mountainous precints that encircled their secluded valley. They are almost wholly a pastoral people, and have about as much idea of the rest of the world, as we have of people in the moon. But notwithstanding their want of mental culture; their mental cabinet seemed full of primitive idea, & shone out in all the simplicity of unsophisticated nature, ameniable only to the few restrictions of conventional propriety. There was a semblance of rustic Aristocracy among the leading men in society, bearing a Quixote gentility, & made significant in the wearing of side arms. The majority however had attained a little more than savage rusticity.

In their dress & demeanor, as uncouth and grotesque as intentioned nature could invent. As an evidence of their barbarism, it may be only necessary to remark that female beauty was considered enhanced when the features become so thoroughly tattoed as to preclude recognition.

On the fourth of July what Americans was in town aided by the French residents, came together with a view to give an expression of national pride by rallying under the proud banner of our country, & going through a few military evolutions. Our display which to them was no doubt quite novel, brought together the whole "posse comitatus"[27] of the place, who fell into procession with "ragtag & bobtail,"[28] & the most grotesque band of music imaginable at their head, alternated with shouts of *"Viva la Republica"* at every halt and corner. The occasion was crowned with two crowded fandango at night, when all the Americans were invited to participate. As for myself I took no part nor yet was I an idle spectator, for I felt that I had been suddenly translated from civilization to barbarism and placed at a stand point no ways unpropicians[29] for to form an estimate of moral rectitude, and especially compare the ostensible religions of the day.

On the 7th July Mr. Beheal [Vigil] the Customhouse officer arrived from Sta Fee [Santa Fe] to assess what goods came by way of Taos. The

[27]*Posse comitatus* in this context is defined as a crowd or rabble. Stanford, *Stanford Dictionary*, 643.
[28]*ragtag and bobtail:* the common people (e.g., the rural residents of Taos).
[29]Willard's meaning is unclear.

Alcade sent for me to bring in my medicines, but I did not heed his mandate chosing to call on the officer proper for direction. I accordingly went into town & got an introduction to him when he informed me I need not bring them in as he could come out to my place of boarding & see them. Accordingly the next day he came out & having learned the probable amt of duty in market that I need not mind the antics, he would pay them himself.

I remained at Taos from the 2 of July to the 15 of September & in the time acquired quite a practice but not having understood the limited extent of Spanish probity, lost nearly all of my charges amounting to some $200.

But the time was not altogether lost to me as I was brought into daily intercourse with them was the better able to acquire their language. Moreover my experience was worth something at least.

At the Ranch [Ranchos de Taos] a village of some 500 inhabitants I got considerable practice & among it an interesting case of "Fungus Humitodes"[30] or bone cancer commencing in the left eye. The patient a man of some forty years of age was anxious that I should do something in his case, & when informed that nothing could be done except to extract the eye, readily consented to the operation. The nature of the disease was not yet fully developed & hense I consented to opperate. I took the eye out clean from the socket, but in dissecting the lower side of the tumour found its base extending down the face riding upon the base of the cheek. I had never before seen a case like it & was a little at a loss what to name it at first. The old man after saying his prayers, invoking the virgins clemency & intercession, sealing the ceremony with repeated crosses sat deliberately down, and like a soldier or a martyr bore it manfully.

The lids or torso of the eye being cut away, I brought the integuments together which adhered kindly, but the excision of the fungii multiplied its legs and it lifted the periosteum of the face & soon made it appearance from under the gums, filling the nose &c. I soon perceived that my efforts would prove abortive & he soon fell a victim to the malady.

Through the request of Mr. Chambers I visited the chief of the

---

[30]Humatodes of the eyeball are a type of cancer. Mason, "Association Intelligence," 125.

Pueblo Indians who was labouring under dropsy. This tribe are in a manner civilized having espoused the Catholic religion, & keeping up the ordinances through the administrations of a Priest who resided with them. This tribe had been at one time a powerful one, & had built a considerable village at the foot of the mountain, but the hostile tribes made war with them & well nigh exterminated them, destroying their houses & greatly damaging all their interests. And in order for self preservation they erect their houses & dwelt in subteranian rooms say from ten to fourteen feet square nicely covered over so as to shed rain leaving a scuttle in the center, giving light & entrance to the domicile, which was plastered with lime mortar & had the appearance of domestic comfort.

In these fortresses the remnant of the tribe could dwell in safety, as no enemy could descend a ladder with impunity, their cabins being well stored with savage munitions. The idea of an underground village was quite novel indeed, but of late years I am told they have been unmolested by their neighbouring tribes & they have again fabricated a little villa above ground. The chief expressed much gratitude for my attentions while his wife spared no pains in preparing for me refreshments. On one of my visits I met with the Priest (a Spaniard) who seemed greatly taken with me & urged that I should stay overnight and seemed quite importunate. He asked many questions relative to geography which I could understand far better than I could answer them. The similarity of language in most technical terms enabled me to comprehend the drift of his discourse, and greatly desired the use of the Spanish tongue to tell him the little I knew of the subject in point. It was not until I urged the necessity of seeing a patient in town that he would in anywise consent that I should leave.

About three weeks after my arrival to Taos, I was sent for by Priest Rada of St. Cruis, 50 miles distant to visit his woman who I found labouring under bronchitis & remained with him a day & two nights for which he paid me $20. Through what means he had learned of me I never knew, but presume it was at Sta Fee through the American company, who I am confident exaggerated my medical qualifications.

I had received a letter from Captain Morris at Santa Fee bearing the Governors compliments wishing me to visit him but I concluded

I would remain at Taos until the American company should leave for Missouri in order to send letters by them & an order for medicines.

Mr. Rennison came to spend a few days with me before starting for Missouri. He had been sick a few days & under my care but was becoming convalescent. The old gentleman professed almost unbounded friendship for me from our first acquaintance & I had not failed to reciprocate kind regards in return, and I had the more effectually touched his sympathies, having presented him with my large fine mare which was worth but little there, & yet valuable in Missouri. I concluded that I would much rather bestow her, than sell at a sacrifice. The old gentlemen was greatly elated, and how to express his gratitude he hardly knew, but concluded that since remuneration was due his old friend, and being a Tailor by trade, concluded no doubt that a benefice might be effected more easily through that medium than any other, and after maturing in his own mind his plan, in his broad "Hinglish" remarked that he wanted to take my measure. The proposition was entirely unexpected to my best knowing it would do him a pleasure consented he should measure, me feeling fully apprised of the wherefore, but asked no questions knowing that so generous a spirit as he ever manifested should not be repulsed. I have only to say, that the next spring's company from Missouri, we entrusted with the present under special charge of safe delivery to his friend the Dr. The suit found its way to Chihuahua through the kindness to the various consignees to whom they had been entrusted.

In reviewing that part of my life, & suming up the routine of unmerited favor which in that country was manifested throughout all my intercourse, I am constrained to recognize the hand of a kind providence which not only preserved my life, but prospered my way & gave me favor in the sight of the people. So far as I know, I was favourably regarded by all, and all were helps while no one hindered.

On the 1st of September [1825] the company from Sta Fee having collected at Taos, concluded to set their faces for home & request me to accompany them into the mountains where they were to organize for the journey. I accordingly wrote a few letters together with an order for a bill of medicines & accompanied them to their place of rendezvous. Esq. Cave was quite ill & was obliged to take medicine. I also administered to several others. I was moreover requested to assist them in organizing the company by electing the officers & arranging the messes. This was done in the evening, as also, a very unpleasant duty growing out of a theft which had been committed some days before, & which was thought someone of the company was guilty. It turned out that a young man by the name of Gayheart[31] was identified as the culprit. He went out in the company I did & I had occasion to see his malice temperament in the treatment of his riding beast a very fine mare which he would fall out with from no apparent cause. I have seen him while riding with rifle in hand try his best to knock her down but she was keen eyed, & I believe invariably dodged his blows.

He was morose in temperament, & uniformly taciturn, having communion with none. The money he had taken belonged to a member of the company, to whom it was returned, whether he was afterwards apprehended I know not. After parting with the company & seeing them off, I returned to town much fatigued having rested but little through the night.

My practice had become tollerable extensive, but as yet I had got comparatively little. Nevertheless thinking the greater portion would be paid, authorized a young friend to make the collection & send them to me & immediately arranged for my journey.

On the 15th of Sept. I left in company with Richard Campbell for Sta Fe calling at Priest Rados & on several other friends reaching the city on the second day at sunset. Señor Vigil the C.H. [customhouse] Officer met me, & insisted I should put up with him expressing great friendship.

I readily accepted his kind invitation, & was soon ushered into the presence of his family. Mrs. Vigil was quite indisposed & I was immediately consulted, not wishing to open my trunks, recommended a domestic application which acted like a charm & thus far my professional dignity was sustained.

It was rumoured the next morning that the American Doctor had arrived. The Governor, Don Manuel Narabona[32] being unwell &

---

[31]William Gayharte [Gayheart] is listed in the Treasury Report Santa Fe 1826–1827. The treasury report shows the transfer of funds of the public treasury from Don Juan Bautista Vigil to Agustin Duran. William Gayheart paid a duty on August 10, 1826, as listed in factura #5, and a William Gayehart [Gayheart] is listed during January 1827. Weber, *Extranjeros*, 18, 25–28.

[32]Dr. Willard is mistaken. Governor Narbona's first name was Antonio.

learning [of] my arrival, sent for me. I visited him in company with Mr. Anderson[33] who acted as interpreter, I administered to his relief paying him several visits during my stay. I also had the pleasure of treating his daughter for an abscess upon the knee pain consequent to a bruise & had become cronic.[34] After I had examined it in presence of her father he inquired if I thought I could do anything for it. I told him that I thought I could & stepped home & got my pocket case & proceeded to introduce a small seaton which discharged the matter at its most depending side. A healthy inflammation was soon excited & did well. The Governor seeing the adroitness with which I dispatched the case turned to my interpreter & said "tell the Doctor that when he leaves that I will give him one of my best mules & moreover letters to the Governor of Chihuahua."

Santa Fee contained at that time about 2,000 inhabitants the major part of them quite poor. It was founded in the beginning of the seventeenth century & I should judge had seen better days, but seemed to be in a state of dilapidation but probably since revived.

I remained at Santa Fee ten days visiting the sick with Dr. Bivires in the day time, while every night a fandango went off attended by most of the Americans. It was "high life down stairs" all the while.

Col. Ward, Dick Campbell, Floid, & Irish Irin[35] the interpreter, got ready to start on the 29th for Sonora while I concluded to accompany them to Carasal, & from there get a passage to Chihuahua. When we were about starting the Governor's Servant came with the mule, & also a letter to Gov. Garcia of Chihuahua.[36] Sr. Vigil likewise gave me letters to his own accord, & we were soon under way passing several little towns at which they sold some goods.

---

[33]Most likely it is William Anderson who accompanies Dr. Willard.

[34]Likely a prepatellar bursitis, which formed an abscess that Dr. Willard lanced.

[35]Ira A. Emmons is listed, along with Dick Campbell, as receiving a guía on September 23, 1825, with their destination listed as Sonora. Weber, *Extranjeros*, 24. Emmons is an Irish surname.

[36]Alejo García Conde (1797–1826) was the father of Francisco G. and Pedro García Conde. Alejo served as military governor of the northwest inland provinces, which included Chihuahua. There are numerous administrative letters from Governor García to Lt. Colonel Facundo Melgares with military orders and appointments in the Spanish Archives of New Mexico. His son Francisco G. would serve as governor of Chihuahua from 1840 to 1842, and Pedro served as general in the Mexican army, member of Congress, and commissioner of the Mexican boundary survey commission. Twitchell, *Spanish Archives of New Mexico*, 632–36; Wilson and Fiske, *Appleton's Cyclopaedia of American Biography*, 2:592.

We arrived at a little town called Toma[37] on the sixth, where we staid overnight calling for supper & lodging. Our meal had to be ground by hand & the miller (a young girl) had been punished I presumed for she was crying over her hand mill sheding tears copiously. But little attention was paid us, and I did not care to wait for supper & lay down among the stuff. In the morning after breakfast the Col. tried to sell the old lady some goods but nothing suited. We then offered to pay our bill & offered her Sand dollars but she utterly refused them. We then sent Irin to inquire of the *Alcalde* if the money was lawful tender, he said it was & that she might take it or go without & we left her & turned back one & half miles to the residence of Ex Governor Baca.[38] The old man seemed pleased at our call, & urged we should stay with him over night. We were made welcome to the best the house offered.

He got me to visit his sister a short distance off and advise her leaving such medicines as I thought she needed. Next morning he ordered a couple of fat sheep dressed & when we offered to pay him, he refused it with disdain. When we came to start we found a servant from the old lady at Tome wishing us to pay him. The interpreter asked him if he had an order from his mistress, & when told he had not, Irin replied, that he did not know him, & the Colonel felt so indignant, that he passed by determined to learn thru a salutary lesson. The money

[37]Tomé, New Mexico, is located about thirty miles south of Albuquerque on State Highway 47. It was named after the first settler, Tomé Dominguez, who had an estancia here before the revolt, probably near the Cerro Tomé, a trail landmark. The Dominguez family left for El Paso del Norte with the balance of the refugees and did not return with de Vargas. Tomé was resettled in about 1740 as a frontier town. Many of the first settlers were *genízaros*, the same class of Christianized Indians that had settled in Ojo Caliente and Abiquiu in northern New Mexico. Tomé was one of the main genízaro settlements of New Mexico in the mid-eighteenth century. Visitors to Tomé included Bishop Tamarón in 1760, who remarked that Tomé was a new town with a "decent church" already built. In one afternoon the bishop confirmed 402 persons while there. Nicolás LaFora, just a few years after Tamarón, noted many changes in the area. He counted seventy residents in Tomé, or the Pueblo of La Limpia Concepcion, as he called it. Pike stayed near what he called "St. Thomas" on March 9, 1807. He reported that the population was five hundred and that the camp was constructed to be able to withstand an attack. Coues, *Expeditions of Zebulon Montgomery Pike*, 628. Due to a shift in the bed of the Río Grande, Dr. Willard would have traveled on the western road through the plaza of Tomé. Jackson, *Following the Royal Road*, 55–56.

[38]The former governor is probably Bartolomé Baca, who served as governor under the administration of the Republic of Mexico from 1823 to 1825.

we offered was good silver coin, but a handsome coin had begun to circulate a little & the old woman thought she would prefer it.

We left the river about 3 P.M. in order to cut off a large bend in the river. Rain insued which turned to snow, moreover night overtook us & it was with difficulty that we kept the road as it was but little travelled. Ward become quite anxious as to our fate & borrowed some trouble lest we should get lost. I got down & led my mule feeling the road with my feet continuing on until at length we heard a dog bark which gave signs of domesticity.

All of my company were in the habit of taking their brandy twice or thrice a day, & at first would offer me the bottle, but I uniformly refused until they ceased to invite me to participate. At this place their brandy was out, and it was with considerable trouble & expense, they obtained more. But have it they must. Ward, who had expressed not a little chagrin & impatience, now became cheerful & even funny as the potent drop necessitated the flaying energies.

It's but a poor soldier that could not hang upon a peg for one night if necessity should require it save he. I thought to myself, that had I have been as impulsive & yet as irresolute, when loosing our way, we might have remained upon the sand plains all night, but the hour of trial had passed, & we were again in the arms of comfort & domestic cheer.

We arrived at El Passo[39] on the 18th of Oct [18]25 where we found some Americans. It is at this point that the present line dividing the Mexican government from our own passes.[40]

It was a place of some 1,000 inhabitants, perhaps, and where a considerable wine & Brandy was made from the grape, which is cultivated somewhat extensively here. Colonel Ward who is rather addicted to card shuffling was easily drawn into a game of Monte with a Spaniard

[39]El Passo is El Paso del Norte or Ciudad Juárez today. El Paso del Norte began as a religious community when the padres established a mission there in 1659. It became a civilian community in 1680 with the influx of Pueblo Revolt refugees. According to Bishop Tamarón, the population was 4,800 in 1760. The population stated by Dr. Willard provides is grossly underestimated, probably in part because he was traveling quickly down El Camino Real.

[40]Dr. Willard wrote this autobiography sometime prior to 1867. By that time the boundary between the United States and Mexico had been established as a result of the Treaty of Guadalupe Hidalgo (1848) and the Gadsden Purchase (1854).

& it was reported he lost the first night $150 but I think he afterwards regained a part of his money ~~back again~~.

After leaving the Passo we came to no more inhabitants until we arrived to Carasal distance 85 miles.[41] We suffered greatly from a protracted cold rain having no tents to shelter us. Two or three of us got into the wagon to screen ourselves from the rain, but the place was too strait for us & I then tried it under the wagon but being quite wet felt but poorly stead with in the morning.[42]

We reached Carasal on the 23d Oct. when my company left me they being bound for Sonora & myself for Chihuahua. They remained here having a day to sell goods & before leaving Mr. Campbell (who could best talk Spanish) engaged a man to take me to Chihuahua & he immediately went for his horses.

After my company had left, I was called on by Don Jose & told to make it my home with him while I staid. I was also visited by several young officers who had charge over a few soldiers probably to keep in awe the surrounding tribes of Indians. At this place was also a dilapidated prison but so far as I now noticed without inmates. I went into there & saw the names of several Americans who had been incarcerated some three years before, they having gone into that country during their struggles for liberty with their mother country & justified their conduct alleging that they were probably spies.

Two of these prisoners (Beard & Chambers) were then living at Taos & with whom I became acquainted. Beard having died the next year of fever.

I remained at Carasal 8 days, when I was unexpectedly called on by a young man who rode up having a horse in leading & who very modestly inquired if I wished to go to Chihuahua & at the same time signifying that I could have the loose horse to ride if I wished him. About that time Don Jose came up & after conversing with him a moment turned to me & said that I had better go with him.

---

[41]The presidio at Carrizal was built in 1773. By the late 1700s about seventy-three soldiers were stationed there. In the 1830s, when Josiah Gregg passed through Carrizal, it had grown to about three to four hundred residents. Jackson, *Following the Royal Road*, 108–109.

[42]Dr. Willard's use of the word "stead" presumably meant he wasn't in good stead due to the rain the previous night.

My mule was feeding in sight which I soon caught. While I was packing my mule, my host brought me a large supply of biscuit & cheese, & we were soon under way. I expressed my gratitude as well as I knew how & being unacquainted with the language, felt circumscribed in my acknowledgements, but supposed it to be my last interview.

The young man & myself sped our way as fast as we could walk continuing until after night & having bright moonlight. I at length signified to him that we had better stop, when he turned aside into the bushes & dismounted. After hobbling our animals we ate a little bread & cheese & then we lay down I having made a couch on which I required him to lay with me feeling myself far safer than to have him lay by himself. I considered that he could not well place himself in an attitude offensive without detection which would afford prompt resistance.

Being quite weary I soon fell asleep, but at midnight I was suddenly aroused by a thundering noise which brought me to my feet. The cause was soon quite apparent, a drove of wild horses had chanced to encounter us which produced what is denominated a "stampede" or furious running of the heard. We ran out & soon found the two horses but the mule was missing. I mounted one of the horses & my man the other in drawers & rode some distance in a search of it, but without success. Before leaving camp I hung up my large Mackana [Mackinaw] that we might be able to find our encampment again. We returned & lay down again until daybreak, when my man caught a horse & put off in great haste & soon returned with my mule which we immediately packed & were on our way. He informed me as near as I could understand, that a caravan was just before us, & sure enough we soon overtook a company of packers bound for Chihuahua to whom the young man belonged. It seemed that they had got word of my lying at Carasal waiting for an opportunity to go down, & sent the young man for me.

We joined their company which I found quite agreeable & kind. On the 6th of Nov. we reached Chihuahua nothing occurring on the way except having my mule stolen at Incinillas. We passed through the village & encamped some mile or two beyond, but someone in the village no doubt fancied her, she being a fine animal. The company detained some 2 hours in search of her, without success, & gave her up furnishing me with two animals instead of one, & I would here remark that in about a year after, my mule was identified by an American friend at the Passo, recovered and sent to me at Chihuahua. The caravan encamped in the public square or "plaza" where I remained with them until after taking some refreshment, when the main man told me he would accompany me to the house of Don Salvadore Porras I having a letter from Sr. Vigil to him. I was accordingly ushered into his presence a dignified old man quite corpulent, & said to be wealthy.

He assured me that his house was mine, & ordered my effects carried to a new house just finished giving me the keys, and at the same time saying that I must eat at his table and consider myself at home.

It may be in order here to describe the city & its inhabitants showing the contrast which obtains among nations. But I had heard some of our company say that it was impossible to know this people without living among them, & the remark is not without might for to know a people, is to dwell with them, & witness the becoming of their entire generation from infancy to age.

The authorities of the City claim a population of ten thousand, the streets are laid out at right angles, & built rather compactly, but it walls resemble mural defences externally a strong gateway & grated windows without glazing but closed by rude shutters. The materials necessary for building consists mostly of poles or beams which support the roof window gratings doors & shutters while all the rest is of the common earth cut up & molded into "adobes" of some 18 inches long 12 inches wide & 6 in thick dried in the sun then laid up with mud mortar & afterwards plastered with lime mortar inside & out. The roofs are of common earth made undulating so as to throw the water into storm spouts which pass through the parapet carrying the water clear from the wall. The roof is thoroughly plastered with lime, mortar & usually proves a safe guard except in heavy protracted rains. Most good residences are built on a square of some hundred feet which is covered with a tier of rooms all round having an inner court or area usually paved with flat stones & entered by a ~~strong~~ gateway which when barred protects the whole premises. The better finished residences have a coridor attached to the inner front of the whole court that a pass may be had from room to room under cover. A portion of these quadrangular rooms are assigned to the domestics out room, Kitchen, & etc. while those facing the streets compose the parlour (*salas*).

The city has a *Parroquia* or parish meeting house constituted wholly of hewn stone and constructed according to the orders, having two massive spires in front, and spacious dome in the rear. The roof is sustained upon pillars & arches & would do honor to a more civilized community. The building is said to have cost $300,000 and raised from a certain percentage tax on the precious metals taken from the mines. The altars are gotten up in considerable task, while the floor is laid with paneled wood, the belfrey's contain four bells of graded tones so as to form a kind of harmonious chime. These bells are in great requisition as but few hours pass unbroken with public announcements of eclesiastical domination.

A religious exterior enshrouds everything, for Catholicism giving hint to every grade & department of society, virtually dying everything as it were in the wool. The altar and the confessionals, are seldom vacated, but are allowed continually occupied by the saint adorers, while the presumptious incumbent essays to shrive them[43] free of actual sin, & ease a conscience made quiescent through false religion & depraved morality.

Added to the *Parroquia* is a Temple dedicated to their patron Saintess called "Guadaloupe." This edifice is not so well got up but presents some splendor especially the internal finish. The dome is high & spacious, giving great effect to the least whisper or voice, which seems to ascend the dome & then rebound in confused reverberations from side to side. Over the altar were carved in stone the four beasts described by John in the apocalyptical vision, resembling the Lion, the calf, the man & the flying eagle.[44] The gallery in front of these beasts is guarded by banisters & railing mostly wrought out of solid stone or marble showing good taste.

---

[43]Willard seems to be describing confessions to the priest by the Catholic parishioners.

[44]This reference to the altar is from the Bible, Revelation 4:5–9. In particular verse 7 states, "The first creature was like a lion, and the second creature like a calf, and the third creature had a face like that of a man, and the fourth creature was like a flying eagle." Stanley, *Life Principle Bible*, 15–16.

This temple is built expressly for the image of the patroness saint which is kept here during the year with the exception of the anniversary days assigned her when she is taken from the temple & carried to the "*Parroquia*" accompanied by a large rabble procession who bow down before her at intervals all the way from temple to church a distance of one mile. This Saintess is considered by them none other than Mary the Mother of Jesus, who they say appeared to the Bishop of the City of Mexico, announcing herself by the name of Guadalupe, & at which time she made her guardianship conditional, & those conditions were, that Temples should be built through the country to her name, which alone would secure her benign supervision.

But to return, I staid with my host some eight or ten days when I removed my boarding taking lodgings with Dr. Longar a French physician who had been in the place some 2 or 3 months. He had a Spaniard & his wife keeping house for him and proposed that I should go in with him bearing half of the expenses. He tried to dissuade me from staying in the city, assuring me that he had not done near as well there, as he had at other places further south. But appearances soon became ominous the current of inquiry ran for the American Doc. Don so & so wants the American Dr. & their election was so apparent that I felt for him & after a week or so left for other boarding & he soon left the country.

The next day after my arrival I steped out and at the door looking up & down street when I saw a man across the way looking through a window & signing to me to cross over. I did so & on steping in recognized an intimate friend & neighbour Otis Peck who had left St. Charles the spring before I did & had been touring South. I found him quite indisposed but convalescent. He was in company with a Mr. Farrel who was there with goods.

On the second day after my arrival I was called on to go before the Governor having a letter to him from Governor Narrabona of Santa Fee. He received me politely & after reading it through an interpreter said that the legislature would convene on the following Thursday, when I would present it to them.

About this time the Measles broke out in the city and my services were soon in full requisition. Calls were frequent from all parts of the city, & through the aid of my interpreter, I was soon in a good business, Dr. Longar to the contrary notwithstanding.

I had not been there long, before I had a cordial invitation by Don Martine Larana[45] to take rooms in his spacious house, situated upon the public square opposite the *Paroquia*. The location was the very best in the city, & I was very happy to accept this proposal.

I soon had my effects collected & arranged in good order having got me a nice *Colchón* (mattress) & Spanish bedstead, table, etc felt quite at home.

My interpreter John Finch was an American who had been in the country nineteen years, & a vicious man no doubt when he went there, had not assumed a stand among them much better than a servant altho he was a tailor by trade & might have done well but for his habits of inebriety. Finch has married a Spanish woman with whom he lived but had no children. He had allowed himself to descend to the lowest serfs in Society, hiding his nakedness with a blanket & aspiring to no higher felicity than present indulgence. He had acquired a good knowledge of their language and upon my reputation was received into the Sanctum of pathological secrecy, & from necessity tolerated for the time by the nobility. But whenever opportunity presented, restraints were thrown off & he would again & again indulge in the intoxicating draught. To render his presence admissible, to the sick room, I was obliged to clothe him decently, doffing his peasant blanket and mistic sandals,[46] while I endearvoured to inspire self respect & national pride in maintainance of his temporary preferment, but it was all in vain, he had made a deliberate election of character, & that was only suited to a baser sphere of life, & that alone could now be his appropriate element. My patience was often tried with him, & at one time so much so, that I utterly spoiled my cane having had occasion to use it in chastisement of his insolence. As for himself, he felt no intolerance to the justice administered, but his wife could not break the indignity, & in the moment of exasperation made a presentment to the municipal authorities, who tenacious of legal dignity, imposed a fine of $20.00. I had however by this time

---

[45]Thought to be Martínez Arana.
[46]Mystique sandals, a type of sandal commonly worn for centuries.

become sufficient master of the Spanish idiom to do without him &
seldom had occasion to call on him thereafter.

On the sixth of Dec 1825 news came from the city of Mexico that
the troops of old Spain had evacuated San Juan Allua it being the
last hold in Spanish America save Cuba. So exhillerating was the
news that illuminations & festivities were ordered by the municipality
& accompanied with rockets etc. etc. These governmental rejoicings
lasted several days giving occasion for all officials both of govern-
ments, city corporate, to appear in their varied uniforms, indicative of
public preferment & pedantic, altho there is no mistake that Spanish
dignitaries can act the "*big man me*" with as good a grace as perhaps
is current in monarchial countries & aristocratic communities. The
Spanish Don enshrouded with his massive & richly trimmed cloak,
makes no ordinary presentment.

This true Spanish etiquette however savory of a kind of pusillanimous dignity, peculiar to their nation, or rather a simpering suavity
which glosses over, and under the occasion passive & consequently
transient & often insincere. Their illuminations were well got up &
for the most part imposing. The Parroquia was particularly splendid.
Its many capitals & pendencies in front, made ample bearings for little
pots or crocks, supplied with tallow & wiking which when lighted up,
gave a most luminous aspect. Nearly all private houses were arrayed
with lights upon the front parapet & altogether I think was but little
inferior to those displayed at Cincinnati; on the occasion of General
Harrison's election.

Added to illuminations were rockets & religious processions & every
species of public rejoicings finished up with three days gaming or
gambling, in the public square. To these games all had a cup rich &
poor, noble & ignoble, & I other than a prostituted society, could have
brought in requisition so many schemes of operation swindle, as was
then exhibited. The games (*chuces*) were tolerated by Special pursuit of
the municipal board of *Alcaldes*. Where ever we find an idle community, we may look for vices in the same proportions as idleness obtains.

The constitution of man, in all its developments from infancy to age,
demonstrate that action mental & physical obtains in every country

& every age of the world, and hense when virtue is out, vice is in, & *vice versa.*

On Dec 9/25 all the officers of State assembled at the Congress Hall (as they term it) for the purpose of acknowledging their federal state constitution by oath. I was invited to witness the ceremony which went off with great éclat & acclamations of *"Viva la republica." "Viva la religion 'catolica.' "Viva la Republica Americana del Norte."* They boasted of having our constitution as a precedent for them with the exception of religious intolerance. The Roman Catholic faith alone should be inculcated in the nation.

From the 2nd day of my arrival, I was getting an increasing practice. My little name began to circulate in the country, and invalids began to come in from almost every quarter. The curate was one of the first to patronize me, & served to look upon me almost as a *"God Send."* I waited on his family through the measles, & afterward on himself in a severe attack of Dispeptic Cachexy[47] becoming greatly emaciated, & intolerant to every kind of food. I treated his case as prescribed by the books, but made no progress for the better. I even went so far as to administer the gastric juice of the beef, but to no advantage as I could discover. At length on one of my visits we were conversing on the subject of diet, & he asked the question what diet I considered the easiest assimilated with the blood or what nutriment was easiest converted into chyme.[48]

I remarked that the milk of women I had heard was the easiest concocted, not thinking it possible for him to avail himself of such a benefice, but the old Gentleman took the hint, & sent for a nurse,[49] & began to experiment upon the suggestion, & soon found his appetite & strength increase. He then sent for another nurse & the two succeeded in fully restoring him to far more than ordinary health & athletisim.

I was greatly surprised to witness the prompt effects of the infant regimen, aided by a few simple pills of operative quality. It was also

---

[47]Dispeptic cachexy is abdominal pain and heartburn. The illness was most likely pancreatitis due to an insufficient enzyme required for digestion.

[48]Chyme is the digestive fluid of the human body.

[49]A wet nurse who could provide breast milk, which would have been more easily digested.

my good luck to suggest a remedy to Dona Severena the mother in law to Genl. Arce,[50] who had become quite cachectic & apparently getting but little or no benefit in the way of medicines, having become somewhat discouraged I chanced to advise her to visit the hot springs some 30 miles distant. The readily approved of the plan. The coach & seven mules in harness besides out riders & mules for change were soon in readiness & when the Genl. his wife & her sister with their Medico composed an escort for the old lady making quite a display of aristocracy. The general & myself staid but one day & two nights & returned to the city.

The Spring was hot & torrentuous belching forth in a rapid murmur, while cold springs were issuing ahead in the immediate vicinity.

The old lady staid some two weeks, when she returned greatly improve by bathing & drinking the waters. I had no means of testing the water as to it[s] component qualities but think it ferrugions & sulphurious.

Dr. Bivins & Mr. Sweeney who passed through here a week or two since & who came into the country the same time I did, returned ~~today~~ from Parral he not being able to practice for want of license. He concludes to return home & offered (me all of his medicines) for forty dollars which I bought.

On the 9th of January 46 [1826] Consul Storrs, Mr. Williams and Mr. Parrish arrives & put up with me. I assisted them in passing their goods through the custom house. Dr. Aitkin & Mr. Stephens arrived on the 13th. My American friends seem to take delight in acting out their independence paying but little attention to the religious flumery which is constantly before our eyes. The host is almost daily out & the contiguity of my office to the church exposes us Americans to it sacrilegious nunnery. The sascerdotal incumbent who fills the sound coach drawn by two mules, fine mules proceeded by boys dressed in white robes & bearing crosses, & these proceeded by a lad who jingles a bell to give notice of the approaching host, demands the undivided attention of all within his vista. Consul Storrs while perambulating the pavement in

[50]José Antonio Arce married Justa Pastor de Uranga in Chihuahua on February 24, 1818.

the enjoyment of his cigar was passed by the host in mock solemnity &
pomp unrecognized by the consul. It was noticed by some of the natives,
who reported the fact to Don Pedro Olivaris. This indifference could
not be brooked even in our Consul, & hense a complaint was made to
me in behalf of this slighted dignity. I mentioned the case to him (the
consul) who regarded it as of but little moment at first, & continued
his course of noncompliance. A few days after another complaint came
to me for similar abuses, alleging that the offenders did not so much as
doff the hat, which would at least have been a sanction of respect, even
should they not kneel. I endeavoured to excuse them, on the ground
of their ignorance in ecclesiastical etiquette.

We had previously been before the Governor with the Consul & his
commission had been translated into Spanish & all would probably
have gone off well but for his noncompliance with their religious customs. I informed Mr. Storrs of renewed allegations, of his persistent
disregard of their customs, and suggested the propriety of conform-
ing to Roman customs when among Romans. He said he was fully
aware that national etiquette demanded it, but that he was so utterly
disgusted with all of their religious flummery, that he could not effect
a simpering so ridiculous. And as he contemplated the subject, he
became more & more excited, & attempted to write to the Governor
on the subject but was prevented through a want of the language, &
finally made up his mind to go home & resign his appointment. He
went home but did not resign however; but after an absence of a year
returned arriving to the City the day after I left it. How the second
visit was received I am unable to say.

The Americans were all cited to appear before the legislature, where
they were all interrogated as to their place of residence, occupation,
business to that country, & the time of their sojourn &c. The consul
had not been long in the city before he took the measles having them
pretty big at first but taking cold relapsed & suffered ultimately quite
a siege of illness.

On entering Chihuahua I saw clearly that society was made up of
servile veneration & scrupulously adhered to by all, from the highest to
the lowest, & to trample upon their religious rights, & disregard their

ceremonious sanctity, was self immolation. For while it would effect no good to them in the way of reform, it would greatly lessen in their view, my own claims to their friendship & sympathies, and paralyze any effort at doing them good. Hense I came to the conclusion that I would not be outdone in polite ettiquette, or religious tollerance, and accordingly made it a rule to engage heartily in any requirement within the walls of the church, with the exception of crossing myself which seemed to me would savior of hypocracy.

I was not required to abjure my own religion, & espouse theirs; but I was normally required to tolerate them, by allowing them the liberty of conscience which I claimed myself so also. Their seremonies were their own; it was not my provision to call them in question, whether they were biblical or whether they were heathen, or apostolic, but grant to them that prerogative. I should under like circumstances claim myself. But the Consul seems to have forgotten the nature of his embassy to negotiate commercial & friendly relations with them, & leave them to the enjoyment of their own religious rites. And hense while I was correct & almost worshiped, he was disregarded & treated with indignity, and I am apt to think that to reverse the circumstances, by bringing them home to our own country, we should claim as much. But the consul to carry out his republican principles to the full extent, so far descended as to go to the public square, & purchase his backload of hay & trudge across the main plaza in front of the Parroquia regardless of the speck of people.

I told him it would not do for me, that the highest dignity in society was mine to maintain, hense it was my prerogative to command the peasantry & in so doing, I did not ill treat them, if I paid them a full compensation for their services. I was confident, that a pusillanimous cronying would no doubt be impolite & utterly subversive of professional success. I therefore laid my claims high, or at least nothing less than equality, in every grade of society in which I was called to move. I endeavoured especially to have the clergy understand that I knew my prerogatives & at the same time respect theirs. Hense on being called to visit a young lady who was supposed to be quite ill, so that the Priest was sent for at the same time to administer the extreme unction, brought us in collision or rather into circumstances when priority might be claimed by either of us, but having arrived a little first thought my claim to be paramount to his. I had begun to deal out medicine when he entered, & was about to give directions when the mother came to me & in a whisper requested me to step out a little until her daughter should confess, I replied that if I went out I should not return & if her daughter wished medicine she must take it then, & commenced putting up my medicine again when she with most [indecipherable word] urged me to give it & at the same time the girl reaching out the hand pulled me over & whispering said that if she could have but one physician she wanted me. I then gave the mother the directions & turning to the silent sub prelate said that he could now procede to confess the lady if they wished, bidding them good night.

Among my first patients was a girl in the family of Padre Escontrillas, which I attended some week or ten days, and also advised his honor. Some months after I sent him a bill of services which he refused to pay, or rather did not pay but found fault with the price. I reported the case to the curate, who said if he did not pay it, he would send his a/c to Durango to the board of Cardinals, & they would compel him to pay it. The priest however learning that I was intent on collecting it, & probably may have been advised by the curate, sent me the amt demanded. Some days consequent I chanced to meet the old man on the public square was in company with several other priests, & to my surprise he advanced to meet me, & with warm expressions of friendship embraced me. I mention this as showing the expediency of asserting at the commencement, claims of equality at least, & by a uniform adherence to an honorable upright course, maintain a dignity which would otherwise be temporary.

I was called February 20/26 to see a patient who had been stabbed by a woman, the knife having pierced his stomach, caused great reaching & consequent prostration. Dr. Lopes was first called & declined doing anything but advised the *Alcalde* to send for me & left. To all appearance the man was near his end, but having succeeded in inducing the viscus, he became calm, & revived in Spirits. He was on my hands forty days, when I discharged him & he went to his painting, for that was his trade.

The woman who committed the deed, was adjudged responsible for my bill & required to pay so much per month out of her earnings until all was paid. I allowed her to pay what she pleased taking no account of the matter but am of opinion she paid the most fit.

I could but admire their summary method of settling disputes & claims of every character, by reference to the President Alcalde, whose prerogative to adjudicate according to the sense of right or wrong, put a final quietus in all matters of claim & misrule, save the more flagrant crimes calling for penal corrections. By such mode of judicature, a protracted course of law, with attendant expenses, & many heart burnings are saved, & consequently for the best for that people "who knowing no law, are judged without law."[51]

Custom requires the Alcalde to serve his year with no other compensation than the dignity his office confers, and not a few aspirants stand ready to make the sacrifice of time, for the sake of the honor, which attends his calling.

My practice in the city had become current, while some called in question my pretentions, or abilities. The Spanish Dr. of liberal education had acquired a large fortune, & was running a silver smelting furnace in the city, was more than willing to pass the practice into my hands, and in many instances disposed of calls, by sending them to me; in fact I was often called in consultation with him after he saw that my practice had gained public tollerance. He had the magnanimity to surrender me the palm in the treatment of Pneumonia, & most inflamatory complaints, discerning as he must have done, my better success in mode of treatment which was early depletory.

I greatly admired his simple honesty, in awarding me all my just due at least. He was a native of Old Spain & had been a good student, but had got behind the times, in his secluded field of practice, having probably paid more attention to the extraction of the precious metals, than to therapeutic agencies. He was deservedly a prominent member of society & especially at having charge of the Hospital which situation

---

[51]Dr. Willard and his wife Elizabeth were devotedly religious; later in their lives they were well read on numerous religious doctrines and both wrote on the subject of theology. This quotation is from chapter 35 of the teachings of Joseph Smith, Jr., on the topic of salvation.

was frequently held out to me in prospect, and had I remained there a little longer I doubt not I should have attained to the incumbency.

From the 23d to the 25th inclusive of March the Saint adorns exhibit the merciful tragedy of Our Lord's crucifixion burial & resurrection. The church & street swarm with the pious rabble. My old friend Priest Anchondo from St. Heronimo gave them a sermon antecedent to the pantomimical display, combined with chant & dirges commemoration of the momentous scenes of Calvary. Altho a mockery, it was not without interest. The Jews & Pharisees were prominent action in the drama, and altogether reflected the great truths of revelation.

Owing to pressure of business, I could not witness but a small part of the ceremonies within the church but could identify its progress as reported by the Evangelists. I saw the Mesiah in imagery taken down from the cross, & placed in the tomb of Joseph.

The Priesthood & Pharisees feigned triumph, while the disciples of Jesus mourned in sadness, their dearest hopes being crushed, & they made the laughing stock of credulity. The streets were the scene of satanic jeer claiming triumph over a rapidly growing set of fanatics. But on the morning of the 3d day at early dawn, the voice of triumph resonnated with acclamations of victory over death.

Many beggars in the streets with trailing ropes which girded their loins, carrying an alms plate & soliciting "*Limosna*" for the mother of Jesus. Some of whom had bared their bodies to the sun & inconsequence had become burned to a blister. One called on me for some prescription, I told him to go naked in the hot sun a while, when he took the hint & put out.[52]

During the entombment a procession was formed & the sepulchre containing the body was born on shoulders also two Angels, one on either side, while a rabble of Pharisees followed in grotesque uniform. They succeeded the Virgin and St. John the evangelist, while many men bearing enormous crosses & other lesser ones, accompanied by priests, friars, Ladies, gentlemen, peasants & not a small proportion

---

[52]This sentence is confusing. I surmise he is trying to tell the patient not to go in the sun so that the fiery heat from the sunburn will be put out.

of musicians. A bower had been erected on the sides of the plaza, having several archways neatly decorated with various inscriptions ~~neatly~~ painted on them, making altogether a magnificent display.

I was frequently importuned to be baptized a Roman Catholic & become a Christian, also to take to myself a "Senorita" & settle among them permanently. I usually put them off by pretending ignorance of their religion, & wishing to become better acquainted with their customs & discipline. They seemed to regard me about perfect with the exception of my heterodoxy, & nonconformity to the true faith and provided I would consent to be baptized they would make for me a great feast etc. Not to trammel myself with such a fantastic religion, would not only be Slavery, but in my own view sacrilegious. The whole fabrication was so vulnerable & baseless, that I could not fail to discover its utter incongruity with bible diction.

On the 12 of May Mr. Vigil the Customhouse Officer at Sta Fee in company with William Scott direct from Missouri who brought me a suit of clothes sent by my old friend Mr. Rennison in consideration of the fine mare presented him at New Mexico. I was glad to see Mr. Vigil who had treated me so politely at Taos & Santa Fee. Mr. Scott was a stranger to me & without recommendation, but I soon found him worthy of my regard. He had come with a view of stoping at Chihuahua & working a while at his trade, he being a Silversmith. He had brought most of his tools for manufacturing spoons, forks & other things, but had the misfortune to lose one mule & its load while crossing from the Arkansas to the Simirone rivers of which I had occasion to notice above. After a short acquaintance with Mr. S. I became interested in him, so far as to fit him up in a shop, where he worked several months mostly in the manufacture of spoons. He was a good worker and deserved encouragement but it is a principle of Spanish policy to encourage native mechanics entirely regardless of any foreign improvement. Lumber at that time was all made with the wedge & broad ax, there being not even a whipsaw in the country at that time. A board hughed out 12 to 15 inches broad & 6 or 8 ft. long was worth $1.50. A Sawmill was established in the southern part of the republic by an American, who was ordered by the Governor to stop it, as it would prove an injury to the poor in as much as it throw them out of employment. Mr. Scott however disposed of his wares pretty readily, but felt an inkling to get along fast & bought some articles of commerce & next to the mines & traded a while, as speculation in that country is the order of the day with Americans.

My venerable host Don Salvadore Porras returned from his hacienda (farm) having received a stroke of ~~the~~ Palsey (Apoplexy) on the way & was immediately hurried back for treatment. I was immediately called when I put him under depletion treatment, & he got better so as to walk out a little, but soon took a relapse and died on the 9th of August 1846 [1826].

On receiving the 2nd stroke became insensible & in the meantime an active Erysipelas[53] appeared up on his right ear & spread rapidly over his face & down upon his throat defying my utmost skill. The Priest was sent for to administer the extreme unction, preparatory to his exit. When I entered he smilingly observed that we had met again, he to cure the soul, & I the body; & at the same time was busy in preparing the Eucharist. I saw that my old friend was in the act of dissolution, & called the attention of the Padre to the fact, when he reached me the wafer upon which he had written something, & requested me to administer & continued to write on as many I think, as a dozen a while. I received them from him, & laid them in the patient's mouth, who I think never swallowed them. I have wondered that a thing so holy as they esteem the Eucharist, should have been committed to one who they must have regarded infidelic. But the case was urgent & to prepare & administer to, in season, I inferred was the reason of his making me a substitute. I had occasion to mention this first while in medical college at Philadelphia to a fellow student from Quebeck, who called in question my veracity, and would give me no credit for my assertion, never the less it was ever so. Sitting as I did at the bedside suggested no doubt the convenience, & moreover I being a favourite of his would tend to assuage the sacrilege.

My understanding was none other than friendly with all the Priests

---

[53]Erysipelas is a superficial infection of the skin found mainly on the face, which typically involves the lymphatic system. Erysipelas is also known as Saint Anthony's Fire, which accurately describes the intensity of this rash. Erysipelas was a feared disease in pre-antibiotic days, most often caused by *streptococcus* bacteria.

& especially with the curate, who expresed great fondness for me often inviting me to participate in innocent recreation with cards. I would sometimes find quite a number of Priests who on entering would rise and salute me cordially, & then insist upon my taking a hand with them for pastimes never offering to gamble. Our conversation was on various subjects; at one time the bible came up, the old curate was telling them that he had heard of a book alphabetically arranged so as to find almost any leading word or portion of scripture but could not recollect the name of it. I readily discovered that it was the Concordance of the Bible that he had reference to & concluded I would make an inquiry at a venture in reference to the name of the book. Having begun to Spanishize English nouns a little inquired "No esta Concordancia mi Padre?" (Is it not a concordance that you have reference to father?) He replied rather enthusiastically "Si, Si. Senior" I was gratified in being able to relieve the old man's difficulty & at the same time place myself in the light of favouristism. It was not unfrequent, that demonstrations of sincere regard were manifested, in the bestowal of various presents as fruits, trinkets, HKfs [handkerchiefs] &c. Governor Narabona presented me with a valuable mule, General Arsa with a fine horse also. Don Abellano presented me a horse at Chihuahua, and Don Manuel Moreno ~~also~~ (likewise) bestowed another beautiful riding animal having a gait much admired then namely a marker which lifted his fore feet quite high & thereby exhibiting great action.

On the eleventh of Sept 26, 1826 news came from the City of Mexico that our Governor Garcia of Chihuahua was there on a visit at that place had demised. His death was much regretted. Don Pedro Armendaris our member in Congress wrote home the facts of his death & also sent his compliments to me. He had served as President Alcalde the year before, & hense I had become well acquainted with him through a business channel & also being his family physician. Through his recommendation at the City, a Cardinal & his lady set out for Chihuahua, in order for to consult, me in reference to her case, but happening to be down at the villa [Valle de] Allende, met them there, where I advised them & they returned. I have greatly wondered at the credability of man, & the latitude of sudden, & often brief celebrity,

& especially its accumulating wake which like that produced by the falling pebble upon the waters smooth surface, agitates far & near. My humble name however would not have reached the city six hundred miles distant had it not been for my friend the Senator, but I felt that his gratuity was uninvited altho, in looking back can but regard myself as having done the very best I know how, & especially, labouring as I did, under many disadvantages, having a limited assortment of medicines & yet a tyro in the languages. But suffice it to say, that but few if any one went to that country before me, who, so far as I can learn, did half as much as I did in a pecuniary point of view.

Isolated as I was from the English world, one might suppose that I would have become homesick, lonely, but correct as I was, by high & low, & at the same time gathering in the "needful" found no place for dispondancy. My mind was always with my business duties, & seldom or never clogged. It is true I would sometimes give way to forebodings & groundless apprehension, knowing that I resided among a people abandoned to almost every species of evil, & held in light estimation that lives of their fellow men, when contrasted with lucre; but demonstrations of personal regard at least were so obvious from those of every sphere, that I was not held in painful endearance, or intimidated in my professional rambles at night. In all my night calls, the messenger was accompanied by a watchman armed for self protection, while I could avail myself of his sworn vigilance to & from my patient.

My office was incarcerated as it were, within the inner court. It could not be reached except by the common "*puerto*" or large gate which was committed to the care of some one of the domestics sleeping contiguous, & hense in my retirement was seldom disturbed save by the ~~downstairs~~ porter.

My practice was almost wholly confined to the City which as I before remarked, was estimated at ten thousand. Saint Heronimo a considerable village 20 miles distant, where I had become some acquainted through some of the first families, who had visited me at Chihuahua, & who on several occasions called me there professionally.

On one occasion, I spent there, (three) days (there), at a feast or a Bullfight occasion. Mr. Stanley a merchant from (& who had lately arrived bringing 8 letters for me mostly from MO.) Missouri accompanied me at this time & as but few comparatively, are acquainted with this simi-barbarous custom, it may not be altogether as interesting to give a cursory outline of their national festival made venerable by antiquity. Lord Byron in his "Childe Harrold" (1st canto) beautiful describes this august assemblage,[54] while he points to the life their gaudy display of Chivalrous deeds.

An amphitheater is erected, with decorated galleries perched high above the arena of unequal conflict. The dons & doñas of noble birth laid claim to seats most elevated, while the peasantry found their sphere in humbler circles below. The *"Matadores"* or Champions took their places within the area or circle below some were mounted on horseback while others with sword and banner promenaded on foot. The audience all being seated ~~had~~ in mute expectations, while the clarion sounded to give signal of full preparation for the barbarous conflict. By order of the president the shrill trumpet announced the introductions of the furious bull. Shouts above & all around arouse his brutal frenzy. The astonished brute looked every way for a door of escape, but finding himself fenced in on every side by a taunting populace strongly environed by protective guards, separating the one from the people. Through these encircling ramparts the Matadores could pass when closely pursued, but the narrow pass precluded the pursuing monster. And while he faced an enemy here, another in his rear with dart or spear, inflict unmerited torture.

A routine of menacing abuse, would at length provide a kind of brutal frenzy, exhibited in his rolling eye & lashing tail, with correspondent bounds of offensive warfare. Horses would sometimes pass in the unsightly conflicts in which feminine sympathies were bartered for sports of grossest guise. At length scenes of carnage clogs. The bull exhausted in his energies, while bleeding at many wounds, & carrying in his enormous neck the barbed darts, amid with straining banners, upon which the name of some affluent don or doñas is inscribed begins

---

[54]*Childe Harold's Pilgrimage* is a lengthy narrative poem in four parts written by Lord Byron, published between 1812 and 1818. The world-weary young man whose travels make up the subject of the poem is seeking new experiences in foreign countries. Verses 71–80 describe a bullfight.

to tire in the unequal ~~conflict~~ combat, when the death signal sounds, and the menacing process changes to that of murderous conflict. The horseman with his lance, aims at thrusting it to the spinal chord near the head, which when successfully aimed sink the victim to the earth. Others are left to the foot, Matadors who with a sword, aim at the jugulars of the neck when universal shouts proclaim a final conquest. The gates are flung open, & in rush a decorated team of chain mules, which hurls the expiring brute from vulgar eyes.

The clown occupies the area, while refreshments are passed around. The band of music relieves the mind long held in anxious suspence or painful sympathies, until another victim is ready, thus continuing to gloat upon cruelties but little removed from savage usage. Fangdangoes usually crown the sport of the day & serve to polish or refine the grosser entertainments of the Amphitheater. But the mind clogs amid all the varied changes of tragic scene, and finite material again relapses into the oblivious state of balmy sleep. The above scenes are usually continual for three days engrossing the time & attention of all classes from the Governor to the lowest serf, comprising whole communities.

On our return to Chihuahua were kindly greeted by the waiting friends, many of whom were importunate medical attentions. Mr. Stanley was quite a gentleman & with myself invited frequently to spend our evenings a broad diverting ourselves with loteria or other innocent games for pastime. On one occasion we visited General Arsa's family, which I had been waiting on some time, the mother in law having been quite indisposed and entertaining ourselves a while, the General asked us how much my bill was I told him that I had made no charge. He steped out, & returned in a few minutes with ~~fifty~~ 100 dollars in silver & threw it into my lap. I exclaimed that it was too much, & gathered up my two hands full, & cast it into the mothers lap, & pocketing the rest. I found it generally best to make no charge in such families, as their sense of honor precluded anything like parsimony. I found many among that people whose magnanimity far exceeded the narrow policy so much met with in the United States. This was exemplified on occasions of visiting places of amusement in company with families' male & female.

The gentleman, who first approached the door, would pay for the whole company. Money stood (in) the guise of subserviency & not of mastery. Its intrinsic value was less estimated than its equivalent in compensation whether of gratification, or mercenary chattle. I never knew of a subscription Ball or entertainment, as the expenses were usually sustained by one, two or three. This custom also obtains among the French of Missouri. In the long evenings of winter after Balls commence it is usual for two or three young ladies to designate (such of) the young gentlemen present, as are considered in honor bound to give the next ball, & they manifest it by pinning upon their bosom, a boquet or artificial rose. This signifying, that they have no objection to a participacy in the dance, & if you please will be your partners.

I could but admire among the Spaniards that general proclivity to pastime & merriment. None so low in the scale of importance, but access could be had to merrymaking crowds, whether clad, or naked. The peasantry usually go with but three garments, coarse shirt, cotton drawers reaching to the knees, & a course woolen blanket and these for the most part filthy. But their religion, elastic as it is, imposes no restraints which cannot be got along with, by doing a little penance or feeding the priest a little, to shrive them free, thus setting at ease a stifled conscience credulously entrusting the picture to the intercession of saints, & the virgin, to whom is committed all beyond the presentation. As spurious as is the Catholic religion, it really seems a blessing to that people, serving as it does to form a universal band of union, & acknowledged by all as authoritative, & paramount to all other considerations ostensibly. Licentiousness of all kinds abounds, & by common consent is tolerated. Smoking, the almost immediate successor to nursing, finds access to all grades of society & much the luxury of the nation.

I find a record in my diary that on the 16th October 1826 two caravans of 130 mules with segars [cigars] were brought into the city, amounting to $96,000 all for the use of the (citizens here) & supposed insufficient for the year. These segars are manufactured by the government, & furnished to all the states except New Mexico, where they took the liberty to raise and manufacture their own, being so isolated as to escape public cognizance but individual culture was prohibited by law.[55] From the raising, manufacturing & sale of tobacco, I was informed their greatest revenue was realized. Taxation there does not obtain advalorem[56] as here in for I heard of no import on real estate or caput tax.[57] An international duty, was laid upon all species of foreign import, & also, on species or bullion exported from state to state, or from the general government. I think they required me to pay two per cent to take my money from state of Chihuahua & then three per cent to get it out of the government, a part of which I smuggled however.

The general government assumes to appoint all functionaries as apothecaries, Lawyers, assayers, custom house officers & even down to retailers of segars. The apothecary shops are all government establishments, & their incumbents well qualified to manage them, they being men of science & graduate to their business. All these functionalities are under Salaries paid by general government.

In the city are public graineries belonging to the State having an agent to purchase all surplus grains & milling it in the small even to a cents worth at a time, that the poor shall not be turned away empty. If I mistake not these are state institutions & probably afford some revinew to the state after paying all expenses. But produce of every description must first be <u>tithed</u> under ecclesiastical regulations, which imposes laws paramount to laws erected by civil legislations. Their first vocation is ostensibly religious. The Priesthood must be sustained & ceremonialy they have pushed its rights & observances to the greatest

---

[55]A 1606 decree from King Philip III of Spain restricted growth of tobacco to a few specific locations, including Cuba, Santo Domingo, Venezuela, and Puerto Rico. Selling tobacco to foreigners carried a punishment of death. By 1614 the king made Seville the tobacco center of the world. In order to prevent a glut, all tobacco grown in the Spanish New World had to be shipped to Seville, which became the world center for cigar production. Seville also saw the beginning of cigarette use in Europe, as beggars gathered tobacco from used cigars and rolled it in paper (*papeletes*). Gene Borio, "The History of Tobacco Part I," historynet.com, http://www.historian.org/bysubject/tobacco1.htm (accessed January 6, 2015).

[56]The phrase *ad valorem* is Latin for "according to value." It refers to a tax based on the assessed value of real estate or personal property. Ad valorem taxes can be property tax or even duty on imported items.

[57]In Roman times the chief source of revenue was the land tax. The land was measured and divided into a certain number of pieces, each of which had to pay the same sum of money as a tax. Such a piece of land was called caput. Therefore this reference seems to be to a land tax rather than a per-head caput tax. Edward Gibbons and William Smith, *The Student's Gibbon: The History of the Decline and Fall of the Roman Empire* (New York, 1857), 142.

possible extravagance. Religions feasts and parochial services seems to engross the greater part of the time as well as (imposing) a heavy tax on all who are pecuniary responsible. Their very vices & fragrant crimes are a combination of religious might & ceremonies even when condemnation obtains, religious prerogatives vested in the clergy are regarded competent to shrive them clear of a judicial hereafter. Religious tyranny is stamped on (every) moral, social & political aspect of all orders, the very etiquette of commonplace intercousse was the garb of religious sanctity, and for the most part a flimsey covering that leaves exposed the sainted demon of self ritchiousness. Such is their religious polity, that anything must mar the semblance of pious intention; even crime, finds a hiding place beneath its sanctimonious foldings. For instance matrimony is denied the Priests, & yet the sanctity of their calling absolves the crime of adultery, & every other species of vice and misrule. The sacerdotal incumbantcy defies suspicion, and claims infallibility as an inherent prerogative, while crimes in the laity may call for expiation with the clergy they cease to become such, & are looked upon with complacency.

But what more could be expected from a corrupt, licentious church, with no connections, but papal rule & priestly dominance.

Instead of the assuring word of inspiration to guide them into all truth, they are taught a host of old wives fables & traditions, & even incantatory illusions to trammel the human intellect, & debase them to the lowest grade of humanity.

The word of God, which is the only luminary that casts its rays into the dark faction instead of being reflected through qualified teachers, is wholly eclipsed & through <u>false</u> teaching unites darkness—forebodings of future wretchedness which is alone made tolerable through human interpositions or assumed prerogatives to shrive the guilty for.

Such is the State of Catholic Mexico, & every other government, when religious intolerance trammels the people, & shuts out gospel light & liberty. Their political safety is as unstable as their religion is baseless; they both totter upon the brink of ruin. Truth has given place to fiction & all must erelong vanish as a vision of the night & he as the things that were.

During my stay in Chihuahua of nearly three years I experienced constant demonstrations of their high regard for my welfare and happiness. Evidence of which were manifested in almost daily presentments of fruits, trinkets, choice dishes got up in extra stile, etc. No less than three horses & one mule were presented gratuitously but what was most grateful to my feelings was universal tollerance in my professional calling, and this was not only expressed at the patient's bed side, but demonstrated through numerous visits entirely complementary at my office. In fact I was obliged to regard myself at least a favorite & sometimes even a prodigy. I sometimes thought I should have been able to claim perfection as a <u>Medico</u> had I condescended to become a <u>Cathlico</u> Christian, but perhaps unfortunately for myself, I maintained my independence in religious matters, as well as that of medicine, of which my pretentions were never called in question, as society had placed her broad seal of sanction upon what they thought wonderful cures. If a stranger ever had cause to be contented & happy, I had. My calling quite lucrative & practice quite pleasant &, knowing that hit or miss approval awaited me. I nevertheless took no advantage of my independence, but endeavored to avail myself of all the appliances through my limited catalogue of medical agencies, to accomplished the greatest amount of good, & thereby confirm my reputation which had arrisen fortuitously & which unsucceeded would necessarily decline and prostrate me on a level with thousands who were well for a time, but through endless ambition, indifferences or dissatisfaction fail, to rise no more.

I don't know but I may indulge in some complacency, while taking up my reminiscences founded on the early part of my professional career, & viewing them as less artful than <u>honest</u>. Very far from being perfect, I nevertheless retained impressions of honest simplicity, which I had early imbibed, & which I apprehend proved an invaluable safeguard in after life. I always deprecated sly artifice, as the great enemy of mankind. It is diabolical in its nature, and emits an unsavory influence when its ebullitions are made manifest. Chicanery in youth uncontrolled or unsubdued, may lead to monstrosities in crime in afterlife. The old adage will ever hold good that "honesty is the best policy."

And as I regard it quite doubtful whether these remarks ever go beyond my own family, I have arrived at nothing more than an unostentatious presentation of facts, & principles pertaining to the writer and his associations with the world, in which he incidentally came into contact. In reviewing his biographical pathway, and tracing the order of segments which make up his experience, it is quite obvious that a protective hand warded off the many deadly shafts, which lay concealed throughout the devious a slippery ways of life. I have ever been conscious of an overruling providence, and in matters of religion quite obsequious & yet practically passive. I felt convinced in my own mind, that what was current for religion in Mexico was but a base counterfeit, & all beyond the claims of honest ignorance, nothing better than "Bogus." The puppet mimicry of artificial saints, & even Saviors, evinces a superficial worship, a servile religion.

But as it is not my purpose to tread on the all important subject at his time, I shall pass to take up the thread of my narrative & while delivering the facts by the way, intersperse, such observations as may grow out of the occasion.

My practice continued quite uniform & lucrative. I find by reference to my diary that I averaged about 20 patients per day & that many of them were from abroad. Quite a number of them were from Allende, Parral, Incinillas, St. Heronimo, San Dolores, One from Durango, One from the City of Mexico and for one I prescribed who lived in Quahuila[58] of Texas some 800 miles distant. It was through the recommendation of Colonel Arzas family that a history of the case was forwarded to me & I prescribed as best I could without seeing the patient. I think it quite questionable, whether there was no other physicians personally acquainted with the patient as well or better qualified to treat the case as myself, but such is the credulity of mankind, that things that are foreign are most appreciated, and the more remote, form is school, the greater the charm.

Don Pedro Guerra[59] called on me after I had retired to bed, wishing

---

[58]Coahuila, which is today adjacent to Texas. "As late as the eighteenth century, this northern state was known as Quaguila. . . . People have found it convenient to spell that name according to their phonetic interpretation of the Indian names. The name is derived from the Coahuilte-cos, an Indian tribe that inhabited northern Coahuila." Torres, *Return to Aztlan*, 30.

[59]Dr. Willard is mistaken. Don Guerra's first name was Pablo.

me to visit his wife in consultation with Dr. Lopes but not thinking him more than ordinary, declined rising & promised to meet Dr. L[opez] in the morning. Accordingly immediately after breakfast he called again when I accompanied him across the square where I was quite disappointed in finding him living in a state of affluence & the owner of a copper mine at El Passo which he was then visiting to a company of Americans.

When I entered through ponderous "Puerto" I was ushered into a room where I found Dr. Lopes in waiting & who after the usual greetings communicated with the history of the ladies case, as also his course of treatment. The man then returned into the patients room, to who I was presented with a Spanish suavity becoming the true Castillian, for such was the Doctor, & also the host, I took my seat at the bedside, felt her pulse, & after proposing some questions to her & the Dr. was not long in making my mind relative to her case. I found that she was under the effects of medicine which was producing temporary more inquietude than did the disease and that a little time would go in reinstating her, but as is too often the case the physician must do something to keep up appearances. I ordered an anodine to compose the nervous system, assuring her that she would soon be better, when the effects of the medicine should have spend its influence. The Doctor fully collaborated my judgment in her case & politely requested me to repeat my visits until convelesence should take place.

I called twice afterwards & found my suggestions verified in her case. A few weeks afterwards I chanced to meet Don Guerra at the curates. He accosted me quite politely, & when I rose to leave, he accompanied me to the gate & waited on me through, & as I was about to leave him, he extended his hand to give me a token of friendly parting [and] left in my hand four five dollar gold pieces.

Such evidence of public confidence, carried with them more intrinsic value, than did the token of regard.

On the 18th of October I received intelligence of the death of James Douglass who had spent some weeks with me at Chihuahua, quite a companionable young man, & one whom I felt a considerable interest but the particulars of his death I now disremember, which death occurred at St. Fee. He was a fellow companion on an expedition to the hot springs in company with Colonel Arza as family & much thought of by them.

On the 28th Mr. Stanley arrived, bringing me 8 letters mostly from the States. It was a meeting of no ordinary character. While at Santa Fe, I became partially acquainted with him, he being a merchant of unblemished character reputation among the Americans made our meeting on my part quite cordial & I felt that the reciprosity was very equally balanced. We met at the custom house he having brought goods with him. We approached each other with the earnestness of two fighting fowls, namely with a hearty Spanish hug, with half Spanish & half English until we have finished up our mungeral [mongrel] ceremony of salutation. When the excitement of the occasion subsided a little we then settled down into our mother tongue.

I believe that anterior to my sojourn at Chihuahua there had but few Americans or English visited it, save Dr. [John] Robinson [1810], General [Zebulon] Pike [1807], Baron [Alexander von] Humboldt [1803] & a few adventurers from Missouri who in the time of this revolutionary struggle with old Spain were apprehended as spies & imprisoned for a considerable length of time. The three first named gentlemen were there prior to that war, & bore the character of *literati* especially Humbolt who made geological & other scientific researches.

Dr. Robinson they told me superintended their public works of masonry to bring the water from a neighboring mountain to the public square where stands this fountain which he also drafted & superintended.

The whole structure was of hughn limestone, I think in a circular form, some 18 or 20 feet diameter, & probably 3 feet high constituting a liberal tank with a pedestal of some 15 ft. high terminating in the form of an obelisk. On the four sides of the obelisk were neatly carved the faces of Lions with open mouths from where issued the pure mountain stream with considerable impetuosity having been conveyed through the city underground. The aqueduct conveying the water was said to have been begun by the Jesuites anterior to their disbandment by the Pope in 1773 or about that time, I also heard of a few other names but who like my interpreter Finch were of so little consequence in the public view that no notice was taken of them.

On the 9th of November [18]26 Messrs Moor, Armstrong, Ramsey, Anderson & Morton arrived from Santa Fee; the three former bring with them a race horse which was bred in Missouri & had been successful in New Mexico in wining several races. They regarded him unequaled by any horse in that country. It was soon rumoured that such a horse was in town & that its owner had brought him for the purpose of trying his speed with their best racers & stood ready to accept a challenge of wager. It was not long before a gentleman from the country who owned a fast horse brot him in & after an interview with the Americans consummated a bet of $2,000 as the main stake. Many side bets were made & a day appointed to decide the matter, which was the January 11, 1827. The track which was but 400 yards long had been cleared of any impediments, and all preparations made for the occasion. The concourse was quite large of men, women and children. As to myself I had taken no part but looked upon the affair as a kind of strife between them & my own countrymen as to whom should carry off the palm[60] & as the time approached the interest seemed to deepen. Don Biscenta [Vicente] called on me one day and remarked that a friend of his had left in his hands $130 to be staked upon the Spanish horse, & wished to know if I would not like to take the bet. I told him I would let him know when we got on the race ground for as yet I had not seen his horse, & As yet, I had not allowed myself to indulge in any species of gambling save shooting or playing for something to drink as in those times in that country was quite customary. The eventful morning at length arrived where a large concourse had convocated some 2 miles out of the city to witness the scene.

When I arrived, I for the first time saw the Spanish horse which was decorated with the little crosses suspending from main & fore top making rather a grotesque appearance; giving a resemblance of *vitium sanctum* or a kind of concomitant of religious vice.

I examined the horse a moment soon making up my mind that I would run no risk in accepting the challenge & promptly said to Don Bissenta that I would take the risk. Mr. Folley standing present requested me to let him take the $30 & myself the $100. I replied, "*very*

---

[60]A palm branch was the symbol of triumph and victory.

well." The horses were then mounted & a protracted effort was made to get an even start, but the distance being quite short an even start was the more important. After a considerable manouervring they made a plunge in which the Am horse got the advantage, & the Spanish rider held up. They again returned to the starting place & again managed to get off about together, but the Alison (as they called the American horse) soon passed his [unknown word] & considered victorious by his owners, who loudly claimed the prize. The Spaniards were not satisfied however & to save collision I steped in between them and expostulated with the Americans to give them an another trial, assuming that we could beat them quite easy. This interference quashed the controversy and another trial was agreed upon. I informed the Spaniards that they might elect their own time & mode of starting & that we would conform to it. They then proposed various signals but none seemed to be descisive, but in the meantime the riders kept figuring until they at length made a lunge the Sp horse geting a little advantage on the start but he did not hold it long for the Allison soon passed him & came out triumphantly. Great shouting & loud applause went up from the multitude in approbation of the Allison.

I then said to all concerned, that we would meet at my office that evening and adjust the stakes & the crowd returned to the city. In the evening my office was full to overflowing, and those who had pledged & lost, were punctual I think to a man in bringing forward the amt staked; now so far as I can recollect having never put into the hands of the third person, except the amt in Bissenta's hands, which was forth coming. The Americans had furnished a little good brandy but soon I think indulged to excess, altho they seem to feel (as sometimes said) their keeping. Through all the racing process, I had quite a promi-nent part to act being the medium through which communications passed from party to party but amid all the strife & excitement, I had no trouble in keeping good order, & assured understanding among them. The utmost decorum & strict humour was envied upon both sides, & taken altogether, I confess I felt no little complacency in contemplating the sequel of the occasion. But what in those may seem justifiable & proper, would under almost any other circumstances keep condemmatory as gambling should never perhaps find a pretex for justification. But the loss or gain was not with me the grand dissidertion, but the gratification of national pride or ambition. I felt my superiority over them in every respect & could not brook a challenge, & especially from the dignified Don Bissenta, who so eager for self renown, that he had solicited my lap dog as a present to the English King in the token of respect. He wished to purchase the animal, but I preferred gratuitous bestowal, whether the dog ever reached his place of destination I know not.

At this time there were some 10–12 Americans in Chihuahua & having had little to busy themselves in, indulged considerable in little games of Quits, Shooting, etc. My business kept me pretty constantly imployed, but occasionally took a hand with them.

I perceive from my diary that one Christmas night they got up a fandango irrespective of any argument I could bring to bear in order to discourage it. I was of the opinion that it would not be tolerated by the better portion of community & utterly refused to participate in the matter. Dr. Aitkin took sides with me & we remained at home alone. Stanley was a gentleman & under almost any other circumstance would have stood aloft from it, but they managed to draw him in, & carried their point. I expostulated with them in the name of self respect, as well as self interest, believing it to be ruinous to my reputation as a man & as a physician. I argue that dignity was my only safeguard and I must maintain it at any sacrifice, in order to secure the countenance of the aristocracy of the city. But they were in the majority, & the arrangements had already been made, and the fandango must go off at any hazard. I told them that they had nothing to losse, or gain, as they were but sojourners there for a few days. But for ought I know, I was located for years, & having a moderate reputation must maintain it. They were joined by a promiscuous crowd of commonality, comprising good bad & indifferent & strangers as they were, could not discriminate between them, & consequently subjecting themselves to great indignity, in the eye of higher community.

Having been repulsed by Dr. A. & myself they concluded to play a trick upon us, & get us through stratigum to honour them with our presence. They got together about 9 in the evening, & concocted this plan. It was to dispatch a young Spaniard to my office with a message that Bill Anderson had got high, (which was his custom) & while in a scuffle with someone, had broken his legs that they wished us to go immediately up & set it. This message was expressed the Spanish language & with so much candor apparent honesty, that my cordiality was enlisted, & we immediately set out for the scene of action, when we came within the atmosphere of the prevailing origins & catching the sound of the hilarious music, we begun to suspect a humbug. I told the Dr. to remain behind & that I should glide stealthily up [to] make my observation, & if I should assertain that we had been duped, I would return without them seeing me. Bill was sailing joyfully through the giddy whirl of a waltz & no harm had befallen him, I immediately evacuated the scout & we got ourselves back to my office undiscovered & smothered the joke in the birth.

My daily vocation tho irksome & labourious, was quite lucritiv and Almost daily accumulating the needful & adding to my pile but I found from certain symptoms that somebody was embezzling it.

After making my round of professional calls in the morning & returned to my office, I observed my bed spread raised in front, & knowing that I had not left it so in the morning, I wondered that it should have been disturbed & as is usual sought a cause; the bed being near a grated window, & shutters open, came to the conclusion that a gust of wind through the window had been the agency that had displaced the covering & without further argument adjusted it, & passed on.

I think that the very next morning on my return as usual, I found my bed cover again in disorder. I was again cited to a reconcile the wherefore, & taking up & viewing my first conclusion to which I had arrived the day before, this course that I had hastily & unphilosophically decided the question. It was obviously clear, that a current of air from my window could not raise the spread, but only move it back & forth leaving it still hanging orderly.

My suspicions immediately arose & the cause no longer in doubt, as my trunk containing my all was under the bed. I immediately hauled it out, & on examination found signs of purloining quite apparent. I had laid by themselves quite a number of large Sand dollars weighing about 1 1/4 dollars[61] each, which I had designed bringing to the states, & I sell to jewelers per weight. The most of this was missing. It then became apparent that someone had provided them silver with false keys suited to both door & trunk, & that something must be done to save my money. I had on occasion of leaving the city a few month previous, made a repository with Don Bissente Bissente[62] but in recalling it, found it deficit eleven dollars, & concluded to be my own banker thereafter. But bolts & bars were of no avail so long as under the control of illegal claimants. My locks were so simple that it was not difficult to forge keys to fit them. I was not long however in devising a remedy. My plan was to wait until late at night & then move my bed & take up a brick of which my room was paved & with an old Spoon burrow a sufficient vault to hold my valuables.

The earth taken out was carefully deposited in the back house, and when the brick was replaced & swept over, no signs of disruption could be discovered. I placed it under my bed lest by trading upon it, the margins which sustained it, might give any. My stratigum succeeded admirably. About once a week I could raise my brick & deposited what I had secreted about my medicines & need no key to secure it. Dr. Aitkin deposited with me some $5,000 in gold & felt his funds quite safe. The next year a French merchant by the name Cucier came to the city, bringing with him a large safe which became my repository.[63] Thereafter until I left, Mr. Cucier brought a large amount of

---

[61]Silver was the monetary standard at this time in the United States. Willard is suggesting he will take it back to the United States where the amount of silver minted in the coin will be more valuable by weight than the monetary exchange.

[62]Vicente de Vicente (1793–?) was one of the many Spaniards issued a passport and expelled from Chihuahua on July 19, 1828. He departed from the port of Veracruz, Mexico, and arrived in New Orleans on the ship named *Monk* on March 19, 1829. Rangel, "Vascos en Chihuahua"; New Orleans passenger lists, 1820–1945, ancestry.com.

[63]Esteban (Stephen) Curcier (ca. 1776–1843) was born in Bordeaux, France. While residing in Philadelphia in 1800, he petitioned to become a U.S. citizen. He married Antonia Beatrix de Tastet in London, England, on August 10, 1815. By the late 1820s Curcier had formed a partnership with Dr. Willard and a Spanish gentleman to lease the Santa Rita copper mines in Silver City, New Mexico. In 1830 Curcier purchased the Hacienda de San Marcos del Saucillo, which the Mexican government had acquired in 1827. Curcier supplied the mining centers of Parral and Chihuahua with hides and meat. Stephen Curcier, Declaration of Intention to become a U.S. Citizen, [Philadelphia], March 21, 1800, National Archives and Records Administration, Naturalization Petitions for the Eastern District of Pennsylvania, 1795–1930, Series M1522, roll 42; Ralph Allen Smith, *Borderlander: The Life of James Kirker, 1793–1852* (Norman: University of Oklahoma Press, 1999), 30.

goods having men and teams imployed, that on his arrival brought him in debt to them & wishing to discharge all except his clerks, he was under the necessity of borrowing from me a thousand dollars to pay them off. I gladly advanced him the money which in a few weeks he was able to return me with thanks. He took rooms contiguous to my office. I found him a gentleman & an agreeable companion.

After he had been doing business a few months, & got some acquainted, we formed a co partnership with a Spanish Don thinking to make a speculation in the purchase of silver ore at the mines from 2 or 3 hundred miles distant & freight it to the city for smelting.

Our contract was to put in a thousand dollars each, & be equal partners in the avails but our Spanish partner was to go to the mines, purchase the mineral & bear his own expenses, as an offset to the thousand dollars furnished by each of us. The money was furnished sometime in the spring and he left for the mines, where he remained until the next February. During his protracted stay, we became apprehensive that he had indulged in gambling & squandered our money, although we had received a considerable proportion of the amt invested in ore sent onto us.

But made up my mind to leave the country sold out my interest to Mr. Cucier at $450 & discount he refusing to allow me more. I was afterward informed by Dr. Aitkin who was there that I had not been gone long from the city, until our partner returned with a large & valuable amt of mineral, making it a fine speculation to them but disastrous to me.

Mssrs. Moore, Ramsay & Armstrong the owners of the Allison having consummated their racing at Chihuahua, came to the conclusion to pass down tor'd [toward] the city of Mexico & obtain other challenges for racing, but the fame of their horse proceeded them, & no one dared risk in opposition.

They proceeded as far as Parral a mining town one hundred miles distant where they sold their horse to some Spaniards for a thousand dollars. The purchasers gathered up their stock of various kinds not having much money after paying for him (their horse) & started with them through the country think to meet with success & perhaps realized a fortune. Moore & Co. having received the money remained there for some time & commenced speculating in mineral. When they left Chihuahua, they felt quite sanguin that there was probably a fortune in their horse provided they had a sufficient capital to bet high, and proposed to me to lend them $500 believing that they could soon refund it with interest. Being a credulous young man & thinking as they did that there was money in this horse counted them out the amt. asked for & they left. It was some weeks before I heard anything from them, till at length news came of their having sold the horse etc. I immediately became a little uneasy fearing that I might [have] been mistaken as to their honesty & especially as most sporting characters are to be regarded suspiciously.

I mentioned the facts to Colonel Arce who advised me to go immediately down & secure myself & at the same time offered me horses and a trusty servant who knew the road across the country which would save quite a distance. I unhesitatingly accepted his kind offer & started I think the next day. We steared our course irrespective of roads occasionally meeting with scattered population tho quite sparse. The second night we travelled sometimes after dark hoping to arrive at a certain ranch, but getting tired & discouraged concluded to stop it being quite dark. We threw ourselves down after hobbling the horses, & slept quietly until morning.

On awaking at daylight found ourselves within a few rods of a house. It being quite early, concluded to travel until we should find other inhabitants before breakfasting.

We arrived at Parral on the 4th day I think, when I put up at Alcade having a letter of recommendation from a gentlemen in Chihuahua. As I lighted from my horse, the Alcade came out & met me quite cordially, observing that he was expecting me, having been written to by the gentleman, to whom I was indebted for the recommendation. I was shown a room with an assurance of a hearty welcome. I had not been there long, before he came into the room with a bottle of brandy, saying that he was aware that no Americans were in the habit of using it. I replied that it was too much the case but as for myself, I would be excused.

After I had refreshed, called on my American friends, who I found well. They apprehended my errand, & without hesitation counted me out my money, saying that for my pains I had had the pleasure of seeing the country. I counted myself fortunate under circumstances to "get my money back." After resting a day, we returned in a round about way by the road home, much fatigued.

Trusting gamblers, might have proved to me a disastrous lesson, & would have resulted as probably, had I not looked after the matter in season. In looking back upon the transaction, I distinctly remember the simple ingenuousness of my heart, having no question in my mind that they might possibly be dishonest; but hitherto I had seen but little of mankind, altho I had traversed a series of wilderness journey, & hitherto but little, exposed to artful intrigue. In travelling associations, there is but little danger of ~~practical~~ fraud, being practiced, in as much as to detection will lead to summary punishment. No members of a caravan can practice dishonesty with impunity, for where there is no law that is statutory, a sense of right & wrong as recognised by the party, will adjust all grievances *sin ceremonia*.

Dr. Aitkin a Scotchman by birth received his degree as Surgeon at London. Came over to Philadelphia I think about the year 1820 when he commenced practice & in [18]20 married Miss Meeker of that city an heiress and by whom he had two children. In her last confinement, she was attacked with periperial fever which proving fatal & left him a widower, with two children which were committed to the care of Mrs. Meeker the grandmother.

The Doctor quite disconsolate concluded to travel to disasipate his grief & remote his mind. He also thought to make his tour profitable and to that end, purchased or perhaps obtained an assortment of dry goods on commission to take with him. He went into Mexico the same spring I did, but in the wagon company. He took his goods to Sonora & from there came to the neighborhood of Chihuahua when he sold out to a few Spaniards under a kind of gambling system namely by the yard. The price per yard I disremember, but the novelty I shall never forget. Broadcloth & tape went at the same price measuring tape & other bundles by bolts laying them lengthwise upon the yardstick so also of cotton Balls, Razors, combs, Hats, caps & etc. In Mexico the gambling propensity predominates in all transactions or rather there is a proclivity that way. & Americans think themselves as shrewd & sagacious as their simi-barbarious neighbours & not willing to brook a challenge & hense it accounts for such a strange phenomenon in the varied rules and regulations of commercial usage. The doctor thought he had got rather the best of the bargain, but agreeing to take this pay partly in money and partly in corn to be delivered at the public granaries proved rather a losing game at last. He arrived at the city Dec. 13/[18]26 where he waited until spring of [18]38 before he could consummate his corn trade & realize his money. Saving but little or nothing to do now occasionally, my companion at the sick bed, but would not offer for practice so long as I held the field. We had become somewhat cronyfied he having taken his bed & board with me in my office, made over society quite pleasant & at length, the impossibility of my going to Durango & letting him into my practice there was discussed, until I came to the conclusion to leave for Durango about the 1st Sept. [18]27.

Mr. Shatzell foreman for Cuscier the French merchant was starting for Vera Cruz for goods, & I came to the conclusion to accompany him as far as Durango leaving Dr. Aitken to fill my place at C[hihuahua].

His wagons were empty going down, & could conveniently carry my effects although I took my fine horse which had been presented me by Colonel Arza. We travelled as far as Villa de Allende where we staid over night. At that place were several living who had been patients of mine at Chihuahua & when they learned that I was in transition for Durango beset me to tarry with them a few months at least assuring me that I could realize $1,000 per month if I would. I consulted with Mr. Shatzell who thought favorably of it, & I at length resolved to do so.

Don Manuell Moreno took me to his house & gave me the best room in it for an office. Don Luis Porras who had been my patient at Chihuahua called on me & offered me a room at his house which he thought would accommodate me best, but it was opposed by Señor Moreno & I declined the invitation. I regarded them both fine men, but the latter was desiring my services in the case of his wife, who had laboured for some year I think or more, under a cronic diarrhea & was anxious to have me do something in her case if possible. The disease had been so protracted that her constitution was undermined & at Christmas following she died. Alliende contained some 2,000 inhabitants who were without a physician & it was not long before it was known that I was among them. Calls both medical and friendly began to multiply, when it got out that the "Medico Americano" had arrived among them and it being the autumn, I had no lack of grapes, figs, &c. during my stay there being sent in daily. I was soon in good practice & in good respite & what was of the most importance, compensation was liberal & prompt. Perhaps my best fee was a gratuitous one or rather offered in advance, of the services.

A gentleman living at Parral 20 miles distant under the care of a Spanish physician became seriously & dangerously ill & desired a consultation, proposed to send for me. Dr. Cozine was living in Parral at the time. But the Spanish Dr. & him could not tollerate each other, & hense a servant was dispatched for me. The messenger first called on Don Fernandes,[64] who accompanied him to my office to negotiate with me in the matter. He asked me whether I could go to Parral & see his friend, and what I would charge for the visit, I assured that whatever was right I was willing to go for . . . Said he will $200 answer? I replied in the affirmation. Well said he here is a confidential servant who brought a horse for you, & if you start soon you can get there before dark. I immediately gathered my necessary medicines & we were soon under way. When we arrived, I found the Doctor in waiting, who gave me a history of his patient, case & treatment. I was then introduced to the patient, who I found much bloated and consequently quite incommoded in the bowels. Taking into consideration the treatment, which I regarded quite tumourous & inefficient concluded to give him a thorough dose of Calomel & Jalup,[65] thinking it would give him prompt relief. The dose was soon

[64]This is probably Claro Fernandez, who, on February 6, 1828, was one of the Spaniards issued a passport to abandon Chihuahua during the expulsion of the Spanish. Rangel, "Vascos en Chihuahua."

[65]Jalup (a Nahuatl word) is a purgative tuberous root of a Mexican plant. More commonly the name refers to a powdered drug prepared from the root by mixing it with resins. Neilson, *Webster's New International Dictionary*, 1326.

administered & being quite wary retired to bed; they called me up in the (night) once or twice, fearing the medicine too severe, but its effects were quite salutary, that in the morning I was able to leave after breakfast. When I proposed starting, the $200 was brought me according to contract & the patient seemed fully satisfied of the treatment.

I remained at [Valle de] Allende three months where I spent my time very agreeably & collecting in the time about $3,000 cash & mules the latter of which I needed for my journey having concluded to go back to Chihuahua.

I accompanied Don Fernandes & family to Santa Cruz some 30 miles distant, where we spent several days during Christmas there having a large circle of acquaintances in that place.

The friends were greatly pleased to see us & everything made to render us happy. Entertainment in various ways seemed specially devised for our benefit. The priest mingled with us in a game of cards for diversion, & was as jolly as any of us. It was proposed that Don Fernandes & myself take a hunt the next morning, before breakfast & the Priest agreed to keep the A.M. dinner[66] in waiting until our return, as mass was to be attended the next morning. Accordingly as soon as it was light a couple of hunting horses were brought up, having been accustomed to being shot off of & we mounted with our *[e] scopeta's*[67] & rode hastily up the creek on beautiful bottom land, & at the creek skirted with bushes. My partner was a little before me & seeing a goose, shot from his horse & killed it. The game keeper who accompanied us road out for the goose while he got off to reload & I at the same time road on. I had not gone far before I came in sight of a prairie woolf which ran a few rods & then stoped suddenly & looked at me exposing himself sidewise. I drawed up & hastily discharged my piece at him he ran a few rods & keeled over. The servant rode up to him & slung his lasso & caught one of his legs I think & came cantering up to us. After reloading we hurried on taking a turn toward home. I next saw an owl sitting in a saplin & shot at him when he sailed off into the bushes as I supposed mortally wounded but had not time to look after him knowing that the Priest was waiting for us. We

---

[66]"A.M. dinner" is probably a reference to lunch.
[67]*Escopeta* is a Spanish word for "shotgun."

galloped home & sprang from our horses & entered the church. There was a large audience collected and a band of musicians with box drums & other martial music, instruments and all conspired to make a show & foster the vanity of priests and people. The next day they collected a few bulls, & entertained us with the favorite sports of their nation.

It seemed that it had been got up on a small scale, & with no object to entertain their guests, of which I happened to be honored some of them. They had no amphitheatre or splendid galleries as at St. Heronimo, nor had they the gaudy trappings to fantastic display but the results were fraught with cruelty & danger. On this occasion a more serious & unsightly result occurred than at the feast at St. Heronimo. I presume that the *Picadores* who fought on horseback were less practiced & consequently unskilled. They had not chased the *toro* long before he made a fatal lunge at a horse & plunged his horn into his abdomen. The poor creature in grate fear of the Bull, & of his rider continued to bear him around the circle, draging his intestines after him, they however released him from farther service & I think cast him & replaced the entrails, but whether he ever got well I know not.

> Such is the sport, that oft invites the Spanish maid,
> And cheers the Spanish swains, who gloat on barbarous deeds
> of fight, and smile at natures's ~~groans~~ pains

Our Christmas week at length concluded & we returned again to Allende and entered upon our daily more.[68]

About this time their Congress passed a law to expell all the native Spaniards from their country, within so many months.[69] My friend

---

[68]Moiré, e.g., pattern.

[69]In Saint Charles, Willard had been a York Rite Mason and passed to the third degree. He was elected junior warden of the Hiram Lodge #3, but there is no evidence he was involved with the Masons while he resided in Mexico.

In 1824 and 1825 Masonic factions began to function as political parties in independent Mexico. Two such parties contested for authority during the first five years of the republic, the Yorkinos (York Rite Masons) and the Escoeses (Scottish Rite Masons). In a governmental conspiracy involving some of the military leaders and Spanish friars, the Yorkinos, whose political platform was to remove the *peninsulares*, swept the congressional election in late 1826; when the new Congress commenced on January 1, 1827, more than half the seats had been won by the Yorkinos. These events led to an expulsion law that passed on December 20, 1827, but was not enforced uniformly throughout Mexico. In Chihuahua some 57 *peninsulares* were

Don Fernandes was identified as also quite a number of others in the place, and feeling as they necessarily would, indignant & vengeful, advised me to leave the country also, saying that there was no security in person or property, the contending parties were constantly vascillating up down & everything looked ominous of anarchy & outrage.

I confess that I felt a good [d]eal shaken in confidence, when I came to learn that old respectable citizens many of whom were quite wealthy & esteemed patterns in society, but for sooth because they happened to be down in a foreign country more liable to banishment.

I soon made up my mind to leave the place, go back to Chihuahua where I had left my money in the iron chest of Mr. Coscier & their look around me a little.[70] I accordingly straitened up my affairs and in company with a Spaniard left for Chihuahua when I arrived about the 10th January 1828. At this place I found Mr. Fultcher who had been out into the various parts of the country with a little outfit of goods, & now on his return to the states by way of Texas having accumilated a thousand dollars which he thought he could double by laying it out in mules & driving them through Texas into the southern states & finally succeeded in convincing me that the speculations would pay I accordingly soon made up my mind to get ready at once & commenced my march homeward. As observed above I sold out my mineral speculation to Mr. Coscier at $450 discount, hired a

---

ordered expelled; another 140 Spaniards were ordered excepted and there were 3 unknown or pending cases for a total of 200. Perhaps more interesting is the occupational breakdown of 108 *peninsulares* and the known occupations of these Spaniards living in Chihuahua:

> Merchants, 45;
> Mine owners, 24;
> Servants, 14;
> Farmers, 12;
> Clergy, 3;
> Military officers suspended, 3;
> Ex-government employees, 3;
> Artisans, 2;
> Professionals, 1;
> Laborers, 1.

Sims, *Expulsion of Mexico's Spaniards*, 7–39.

[70] This awkward phrase apparently refers to Dr. Willard gathering up his belongings and looking around for items to pack in preparation for leaving Chihuahua and returning to the United States.

couple servants,[71] bought pack saddles &c & by the 22nd of January [18]28 bid farewell to Chihuahua full of hope & anxiety to see again my native land. Before I could leave the state the law obliged me to pay a duty of two per cents on my money[72] where I was entitled to a *Guía* or passport which allowed the transport of so much money, the assistance of two *Mosas* (Servants) 3 *Armas de Fuego* (fire arms) & thus none should hinder my onward progress, but rather assist me in aught I might stand in need of.

With these preparations, I left the city with about $7,000 cash & outfit, the most of which I had gathered in about 32 months besides my loss on minerals & expenses.

We travelled some 15 or 20 miles & encamped in open country, I started with 3 fine horses, & 3 mules. Mr. Fletcher I think had but one mule. At our first encampment, my best horse was stolen, but at the time I supposed he had strayed back to town & hense dispatched 2 servts for him, but they returned without him. The next day I sent Penilla my Spanish Servt to Doloris he having been raised there but without success.

During my waiting 2 days, I received 8 letters from Chihuahua which Consul Storrs had brought from the states & sent there by my servants which compensated me for waiting.

As we were about to leave a Spaniard road up & inquired if I had found my horse yet, I told him I had not. He said he thought he knew where he was & if I would produce him for four dollars I paid him the amt. he was soon forth coming. I afterwards became convinced that he had been hid out on purpose to get the horse for nothing or a good fee for finding him. Hitherto I had been but little exposed to their thievish tricks, having travelled to Chihuahua in company with caravan, although on that occasion, I lost my mule which I did not recover until a year afterwards. But in looking back I can now say that I was altogether too credulous, but before I got to the coast I became better indoctrinated into the misteries of Spanish villainy.

---

[71]Dr. Willard paid $30 for two servants to accompany him from Chihuahua to the Gulf Coast. See his account book in appendix 2, January 22, 1828.

[72]According to his account book, Dr. Willard paid $80 duty on $4,000 at 2 percent.

On the 26 we arrived at the St. Pablo 60 miles from Chi[huahu]a where I bought a horse and mule, the former for seven dollars, & the latter for twelve. The next day we travelled twenty five miles & camped in open country near the river "Conchez." We travelled in quietly passing don Antonio Palacio's [H]Acienda (Farms) [and] also Santa Rosalia meeting with nothing of note until the night of the 30 when the horse I bought for Mr. F. was missing in the morning. We detained some half day to make search for him but could not be found. Believing him to be stolen gave up search & proceeded to the ranch of the widow Abellano whose husband I had treated for dispepsey with good success that he became corpulent, but he returned to his cups, & relapse again & finally died on my hands, at the Villa Allende, where he had followed me, I first having treated him at Chihua[hua]. The old lady seemed quite glad to see me, & entertained me (with) great Feast, and when I came to leave she loaded me with provisions for the road, & utterly refused compensation. On the 1st Feby we passed Don Augustus Cordera's ranch occupied by his brother. By some means, he ascertained who I was and insisted that we should stop to breakfast to which we gladly complied. I had seen his brother at Allende he having a Daughter living there & married to Don Roberto Morano. Men of distinction are known in that country at a great distance, the population being quite sparce makes what there is, more prominent.

Above I mentioned having bought a horse and a mule at St. Pablo. They were offered very cheap but as it afterwards turned out, proved dear enough in the end. The horse I bought of them was stolen a few nights afterwards no doubt by the visitors altho I did not suspect them at the time. These young men (two Brothers) started soon after we did from St. Pablo overtook & passed us several times accosting as friendly as they met us, and pretended that they were going to Palayo to get a sister, living there. Five days after I purchased of them, the mule & horse, they rode up to our encampment after dark & very politely begged the privilege of sleeping near our fire, which I readily granted. They soon had their horses hobbled when they spread out their blankets & laid down; being quite weary I slept quite sound, the two servants were out with the animals & nothing disturbed us until brake of day at which time I was awoke by the click of a girth buckle. I immediately arose up when one of the brothers accosted me in Spanish "Buena maña [manana] Señor como passa un bien noche." Good morning sir, how did you pass the night? Very well I replied, what said I, are you going? yes said he it's a going to be warm today & we thought we would get along to the spring in the cool of the morning & immediately bid me good morning remarking that we would meet at Palaio.

Hitherto his Bro. was sitting upon his horse at some distance with a large Mackana [Mackinaw] Blanket over him & neither said good morn back. I ordered the animals brought up & breakfast made ready that we might get off early. We commenced packing & all at once I then missed my large pack bags, containing all my clothes, I at first thought they might have been put on & covered over & had them examined, but they were not there. It then struck me forcibly, that the Bro. sitting at a distance was brooding my bags under his large blanket having purloined them through the night. I mounted my large horse Larry & put him under a gallop leaving the caravan to come on leisurely. I galloped my horse 12 miles to the spring expecting to overtake them all the way. When I arrived at the spring, I met an *attajo* or caravan, of whom I inquired if they had seen two young men pass there and at the same time giving them a description of them, *no ha[n] pasado aqui, Nos han revueltado por otro lado, senor.* [They have not passed here, they have returned back another way, Sir]. I immediately discovered that they understood the game much better than I did and that I had been completely duped, & then they had been following me five days for no other purpose then to rob me & to detain them in the wilderness & go back and hunt out the rascals would cost more than my clothes would come to, & so continued on our way.

Until this time, I had been quite unsuspecting. These young men had no doubt been figuring & planning for five days to avail themselves of booty. The boys said that one of them was out among our animals in the night their they did not at that time suspect him of evil intention. But I now regard John who saw their manuvering, to be no better than they were, nothing but cowardice kept him from playing the same game. There had been accompanying us some three

or four days a young Spaniard who said that he lived at Santa Rosal-
lia [de Camargo] with his widowed mother & was on a short journey
of business & after travelling with us a short time proposed to sell
me his mule saying that he needed the money, & offered it quite low.
He seemed to be a discreet young man of but few words, & rendered
assistance in packing & unpacking while I boarded him in the time. In
the afternoon of the day in which my clothes were stollen, one of the
packs got disordered & he & Penilla stoped to adjust it, he being on
foot at the time, after it was righted Penilla being on horseback came
on with the mule, & soon overtook us, but the young man remained
behind & I saw him no more. By this time I began to suspect mis-
chief, & my suspicions began to wt[73] upon the young man, that his
designs were not altogether honest and as we had bought a horse at
Saint Pablo which was a few nights after stolen by the same man of
whom I had purchased began to suspect a similar game in this case &
it being nearly night when the young man left me, was apprehensive
that he would lurk behind a little & mock my plan of encampment &
where all should get assleep purloin one or more of the animals. I told
the boys that they might stay by the "stuff" & that I would guard the
animals that night myself, and to rendered ourselves more secure. We
turned out into a thicket & provided some distance before encamping.
We made a little fire to cook from supplies and then extinguished it
least our place of retreat should be discovered. After supper I took
my mackinaw went out, & found horse & mules all present where I
threw myself down among them & drift to sleep with the charge on
my mind that I was guarding the animals in person & hense found it
no task to wake frequently through the night & examine that all was
safe & then lay down again. At the camp all was in charge of Mr. F. in
whom I had confidence but had I then known the characters of John as
it afterwards developed I might have been more concerned about my
money than the stock. But morning came & all was well. Breakfast
was soon ready & eaten & we on our way. It was now as near as we
could learn, some 8 or 10 miles to Palayo to which we arrived at 10

---

[73]Abbreviation for "weight," as in "my suspicions began to rest on . . ."

ock. & being fatigued, concluded to remain that day for the purpose of purchasing mules which project I had not abandoned. Several mules were brought but held so high that I bought none. I had occasion to remark to the Alcalde with whom I put up that I had bought a mule in few days before for $12 said they could not be got so low in that place. The next morning when the animals were brought up I pointed him to the mule I had bought so low of the young man I had left in the road, he gazed at it a moment when he remarked that the reason he had sold it so cheap was that it had stolen it & showed me the brand saying it belonged to Don Roberto Moreno with whom I had been acquainted at Allende. I saw the brand was his initials & did not doubt the fact. He furthermore remarked that he had been specially requested to deliver all animals wearing that brand & that it would be his duty to do so in this case also. I told him that it might be that the young man of whom I bought the mules had stolen it, but I had said I had paid my money for it & thought I had a permanent claim and should keep the mule. He however rather persisted in detaining it & by this time John came up saying that they had packed all the mules save the one in dispute what should he do with that; put his pack on said I and at the same time pointing to my pistols saying that if he undertook it to detain the mule he would have them to contend with "O take him, take him said he" & never mind.

This slight altercation tended to frustrate my mind some and the consequence was that I forgot my cloak which had been given me by my old host don Salvadore Porras of Chihuahua & hense I thought much of it, & moreover I needed it night & morning. I did not miss it until the middle of the afternoon when I happened to look behind me, saw that it had been omitted to be nailed on as usual to the saddle. I told Penilla to turn back immediately & not to spare Larry, but push him through & that we would encamp early not far from the well.

He whirled back under full gallop & shure enough a little after dark he returned with my cloak. I had feared that he might have been refused but the Alcalde gave it up peacibly.

That night John had a chill & some fever & did not go out with the animals & they were left alone until Penilla came. At his arrival I took larry & led him out some fifteen or twenty rods & made him fast by his *cabresto* or long rope to a honey suckle bush & returned to the fire & lay down again, Penilla eat his supper & then went out to find the animals it being now quite dark. He passed by where he saw me lead larry on his way to find the next, but not seeing the horse came back and inquired when I had tied him. Can you not find him said I, he replied that he did not see him where he supposed I had hitched him. I jumped up & went to the place [I] had fastened him but he was not there. I felt about the bush for the halter or rope & it all was clear that someone had fancied larry & followed me thither & I presumed that the villain was none other than the young man whom we left standing in the road after accompanying me several days. A caravan had just arrived at the well from the east and were then encamping. Penilla & myself concluded we would go to them and inquire if the horse might not have got away & gone to their camp. They said they had seen nothing of him. I was convinced that he was stolen & told Penilla to go & take care of the rest that a search for him would be unvailing.

The next day we arrived at Mapimi about sunset where we kept our beasts buying food for them. By this time the boys became quite apprehensive of continued deprivations & thought an additional servant or two would add to our safety & hense I remained all the next day with the express intent to obtain another or two confidential servants. When I got to the town I inquired for one of their best, and most influential men & I was taken to a gentleman of the name of Manuel Uriste Ochoa formerly from Old Spain who recd me very politely indeed. I made known my business as wanting to obtain another svt. & not being acquainted in the place would feel oblige[d] to him for any assistance he could rendor me.

He observed that all his confidencial servants had accompanied his brother to Durango & would be gone several days. The word went out and that a svt was needed & they soon began to come to don Manuel & offer their services. They were uniformly told that they were not needed, or that I was supplied &c, until he finally told them that I better go with what I had than risk myself with those who would take my life, before I should reach the coast.

I then told the boys that we would start & so soon as might find a man that could be entrusted I would hire him.

My friend Don Manuel kindly offered me a letter of introduction to his friend Don Lorenzo residing near Parral & after laying in provisions for the road & taking directions of my friend relative to the road we left. It might be well here to remark that most of the country through which we have travelled the last five days is quite broken & arid. Mapimi is a small filthy villiage but contained eight silver smelting furnaces all worked by Europeans, my friend was one [of] them & had become wealthy at the business, but the law of expelsion broke up business, divided families & proved to be a great calamity to exiles whether rich or poor although the former had the advantage being able to pay their way, but the poor were to be pitied indeed. We did not get away until eleven but were able to reach the well at dark. At this place we found a few huts, with families who lived by drawing water for caravans. We got our animals watered & sent them to grass. The next morning we got off in good season & arrived at 3 P.M. to the river Nassas which we found high & which we were obliged to cross in a Perogue or large canoe. The ferryman wanted $6 a load, but I told him that I would give him four dollars for crossing all the loads & swim the animals, to which he agreed. The mules were soon unpacked & we shoved off the following the animals & arrived safe upon the other shore. At his juncture a heavy wind arose & the beach being lose & sandy filled the air with dust we hurried as fast as possible in order to get on to grass which they said was a league or two from the river. In being cloudy it became dark suddenly & we found ourselves in the woods with nothing to guide us save a foot path.

I put Penilla ahead with strict orders to keep the road if possible but in the event of geting into the brush to cry out immediately that the loose pack mules might be caught & secured as there was great danger of losing mule and load, provided they should get a rod or two into the brush amid the roar of the wind & the fall of rain which pored down for a short time in good earnest. We proceeded perhaps a mile when our pilot missed his path & giving the signal we all dismounted & caught the lose mules & tied them to the saplins concluding it impractical to get out of the woods until the morning. The poor things were quite importunate for food & continuing restless till morning. At daybrake I sent John forward a mile or two in search of grasses but finding none we packed & pushed forward thinking to find pasture every hour. About 2 P.M. I discovered a cabbin from which a smoke issued when my spirits revived thinking we were drawing near the land of the living & sure enough we found an old man & his two small sons who had struck a fire to cook a little being but sojourners for a few moments. Of him we learned our whereabouts. I inquired if there were any inhabitants in these parts, or whether there was any grass on the road which he answered in the negative. I found we had missed our road & struck into a crop wrought wholly destitute of anything for man or beast & that we could not reach inhabitants until near night the next day.

At this cabin we turned the animals loose & thinking they might brows a little there being a kind of honey locust brush there. But they ran hither thither finding nothing they could or would eat. I ordered them repacked again & pressed forward until after dark where we tied up again. When we ascertained our condition Mr. F. became quite impatient & cast upon me as I thought, unmerited censure. He said that I took everything upon myself & rushed forward unadvisedly & hense our dilemma. I told him that I should not retort or be offended say what he would, but that I had done the very best I knew how; that I had inquired at the river about the road & grass & distance to it but we had got belated & lost or left the road we should have taken, & matters were just as they were, & we must get out of our difficulty the (best) & soonest we could.

He soon became reconciled again & we journeyed on quite comfortably having plenty f[or] ourselves but constantly sympathizing with the poor beasts.

About 3 o'clock on the 3d day we reached inhabitants & after getting something to eat the boys went with the animals to a league to grass. I was surprised to find how well they could travel, none seemed to lag & the longer they went without eating the less eager they seemed to be for food. At that place we remained the next day in order to recruit them a little.

The day following we proceeded onto San Lorenzo arriving a little before sunset. Having gone forward I arrived sometime before the rest & presented my letter of introduction & was kindly received. A cup of chocolate was soon ordered & every attention paid me that is due a noble man. The company soon arrived and provided for with plenty of straw & corn the latter of which I paid him for but for the straw he would take nothing. I remained there two nights & one day to refresh the animal. My baggage was put into a room used for a day school getting out our lunch we all made a cold supper but gave my friend F. no invitation. I remarked to him that I had been eating with the rest & he would make my excuse to his master prefering not to go in. The man went back & soon returned with full rations for us all, we ate a sufficiently & he carried back the dishes but was gone but a few minutes until he returned with a bottle of wine. We participated in that also when he bade us "buenas noches señores" & we went to sleep.

Early in the morning a cup of chocklet & biscuit was sent me & some hour after I was called to breakfast I felt chagrined that Mr. F. should not have been invited also, but did not feel authorized to superceede his sivility. Mr. F. however saw my predicament & gladly excused me. I took John & rode up to Parras a legue distance in order to lay in provisions for a few days. I found it a considerable village comprising a considerable aggriculture or rather worthy horticulture the grape being a staple article, of which they make wine & Brandies. While there John managed to get a drum but I failed not to notice it, and especially as he had forfeited his place according to contract namely to leave him whereever & whenever he should get intoxicated on the road.

The St. Lorenzo plantation was quite large & imploys some 200 hands the year round and was the property of a young widow but at that time was managed by a brother of her husband. I was greatly interested while witnessing the system of management. The labourers were in companies of some 25 overseers or corporals, who took supervision of their work. At night every man was reported or the roll was called & answer given to every name and a strait mark of affirmative, or cross signifying a negation of service. The most of the plantation was in vineyard. I estimated its area to be some 250 acres which was kept clean & well trimed.

The dwelling house was laid out on a large scale, & with ~~grass~~ great regularity, being [quad]rangular. The square was then subdivided at right angles by continued blocks or rooms most of them finished in good Spanish taste. A portion [was] devoted to a *parroquia* or church. Thru the out buildings for the Peasantry in addition gave it quite a village aspect & said to comprise a population of six hundred souls. A school was kept in one appartment which was under the supervision of the Priest, & to all appearance systimatic comfort dwelt there. Everything had a place or sphere, & seemed to be occupied by rule. I little thought that I should ever meet my host in the United States but it so turned out that the next year [18]29 I chanced to meet both Don Lorenzo Don [Jose] Manuel Uriste ochoa[74] & his brother in the city of Cincinnati. The meeting was quite unexpected, but welcome. I had duly appreciated their kindness when in the their country but could not reciprocate their favors at that time, but now that tables were turned & I had the pleasure of offering them my services in aught that I could as for them. They seemed quite glad to meet with me and I had the pleasure of assisting Don Manuel in various business for some three or four years he having bought property in the City & built a house. Don Lorenzo & the other brother returned in about a year to Mexico hense they had been expatriated.

That law of expression bore heavily on many of them, and especially as government exacted duties on all money or bullion exported. I was told at Monterey that an old Spaniard had passed there a few days before on his way to the coast having an *attajo* of mules some of which had pack saddles on without any apparent loading & yet the mules seemed to walk heavily. It was noticed by the custom house officer at that place in & the mules was taken into custody & on lifting the saddles they were found to be quite heavy. They were disemboweled of

---

[74]This could be Captain José Manual Ochoa, commander of Janos. José Manual Ochoa invested in the copper mines when Lt. Colonel José Manuel Carrasco first developed the copper mines in the area now known as Santa Rita near Silver City, New Mexico. Lundwall, *Copper Mining in Santa Rita*, 21–26.

a large sum of gold which had been carefully stowed away there fore safe keeping. The export duty was I think three per ct. or so.

We left Don Lorenzo on the 16th Feb. & went passed Tulagalena a small place when we paid about $1.50 pr. bushel for corn & 25 cts pr. cent for straw & water. This part of the country we found quite ruff & rocky we however made about 20 miles & came to Macuyu 20 ms the distance we passed Patos where the overseers of the English plantations resided. He very politely argued our tarry until tomorrow but Mr. F. thought we had lost so much time, that it was expedient to go on to which I readily conceeded.

We arrived to Saltillo at dark, often passing over some rugged summits with but a mere trace for pack mules. On entering the city I was recognized as a foreigner by a gentleman who addressed me & at the same time directed a servant to accompany us to the Mason (Hotel) where we delivered a room for a small compensation pr. day which was furnished with a table & a few board settees or "bancos." The gentleman who had accosted us in the street was an Italian by birth by the name of Jose Rosi & made great pretentions of friendship for all Americans passing that way. When he found that we would remain the next day he sent a servant with our invitation to dine with him at precisely 2 provided he could get fish for dinner, it being Friday was not lawful to eat meat. He succeeded in finding fish & I was again advised that we would be expected at 12. A Mr. Miller recently from New York was merchandising in the place who was also invited to dine with us. It approximated nearest an American table of any I had yet met with in the country. It was now the 20th of Feb. but various vegitables were on the table as collyflower salad &c. The repast was concluded in the participation of excellent wine served up in "Alameda Italiano." Satillo contained at that time some 8 or 9000 inhabitants, rather better built than Chihuahua; is surrounded by mountain having but a narrow pass out through what they call a cañon. The valley is quite arable & fertile & the city nears the semblance of aristocracy. I greatly admired the suburbs with their rich plats of green and delicious fruits, also the peasantry bore the aspect of comfort, & cleanliness. I noticed several things in blossom, flaxes, peas & c.

I was informed that the house of Bearing & Sons (England) owes all of the country laying between this place & Parras & for which his is obligated to pay a little short of $1,000,000 but at that time had paid one hundred thousand dollars & refused further payment consequent to defect of title. The purchase was said to contain some 16,000 square miles. In the valley of Saltillo we passed a field of some 1,000 acres of wheat having a strait wall which I estimated at three miles in length. We left on the 22[nd] & proceeded as far as Rinconada (corner) which was situated within the can[y]on 12 ms. from Saltillo. The next 18 miles was destitute of grass & water, we therefore remained at Rinconada a day to recruit the animals & the day following proceeded to Santa Catarina 18 miles where we staid over night.

The next morning being Sunday we deferred our start until after mass as they regarded it sacrareligious to start before, but as [it] was but twelve miles to Monterey we did not hurry.

Monterey contained they supposed 9,000 population & rather better built perhapse than Saltillio or Chihuahua. We found there three or four Americans one of which (Mr. Adams) wished to accompany us to Matimoras. At this place I saw orange trees laden with fruit which I presume must have grown the year before. I was invited to partake of what I wished.

At this place we were told the customhouse officer spoken of above might think it his duty to examine our pasports and plunder, & possibly subject us to confiscation, as we had not paid on but a part of our specie. I don't know that I should have thought of it, but for Mr. F who became quite uneasy lest he being caught might suffer loss. We accordingly rendered a strict account & paid balance due. Our timidity cost me thirty five doll. Mr. F. had but $1,000 to pay on, but it was his all.

At this place Genl. Gutieres formerly Governor of Tamaulipas called to see me, I made himself quite social. He gave me a full account of the Emperor Don Iturbide['s] short but brilliant reign which was about as follows. Iturbide was a brave officer under the government of Old Spain and being entrusted with government funds with which he started to Veracrus in order for a shipment, came to the conclusions to turn traitor to his king & appropriate the public funds in his hands to the raising of soldiery to revolutionize the country. His powers was short & brilliant & led to his accession to a limited monarchy, a[nd] finally to a supreme dictatorship. He was crowned Emperor of Mexico on the 21 of July 1822. The occasion was fully detailed to me by Genl. Mariano Arrista[75] who at that time was commander in chief of the Mexican troops, & of whom I may have occasion to remark hereafter.

Iturbide was thrown up suddenly, & fell as sudden. In his short reign several laws were enacted under his decree or sanction, but at his fall, were all abrogated, save the grant to Stephen Austin for the colonization of Texas. This alone survived the reach of his acts.

On the 2nd Decr. Genl. Santana commanding at Varacruz raised the standard of opposition & published his *"Plana"* to reorganize the Congress, & by degrees won over the soldiery, while the better in forward began to speak of the Emperor as a Usurper.

Iturbide began to discover his growing unpopularity & appointed commissions to treat with the contending party. Nicholas Bravo, Guadalupe Victoria, Pedro Celestin a Negretta, & Jose Mariano Michel-and were appointed by Congress as super numeraries & declared that the coronation of Iturbide was an act of *violence*, and that all acts & titles emulating from him mere null.

They thereupon decreed that he should be banished from the country forever but assigned him a salary of $25,000 annually (provided he would reside in Italy & $8,000 a year for his widow after his demise. He accordingly sent in his abdocations Apr 30/1823 & was escorted by Genl. Bravo to Antigua near Vera Cruz where he was embarked on the 11th of May on board an English vessel for Italy.

---

[75]General Mariano Arrista (1802–55) was born at the city of San Luis Potosí, Mexico, on July 26, 1802. He entered the army as a cadet in the Puebla regiment about 1819 and rose to the rank of brigadier general. After an unsuccessful *pronunciamento* in favor of Centralism in 1833, he went in exile to the United States until he was repatriated and reinstated in the army in 1836. He served on the Supreme Tribunal of War and in the Supreme Military Court and in 1839 was made commandant general of Tamaulipas and general of the Mexican Army of the North. In that capacity he defeated the movement to establish the Republic of the Río Grande in northern Tamaulipas in 1840. In January 1851 he was declared by the Mexican Congress the constitutional president of Mexico. He resigned in January 1853, was forced into exile, and died near Lisbon, Portugal, in 1855. "Arista, Mariano," Texas State Historical Association, http://www.tshaonline.org/handbook/online/articles/faro4 (accessed April 11, 2014).

From Italy he proceeded to London, where he took passage for Mexico, came to Tampico near Soto Marina, where the vessel cast anchor.

Here he found that Genl. Garcia was in command of a few government troops which were stationed at that place. He accordingly sent an ambassador to inquire of Genl. Garcia, if he would put him in command of the troops there & join him in again revolutionizing the country. The proposition was accepted, & he accordingly landed July 14th 1824. Garcia put him in command and feigningly went forward to raise volunteers to recruit the army. Garcia proceeded into Tamaulipas and held a counsel with them. Genl. Gutieres who was then governor of that state (in connection with the Territory of new Lion) who joined him sallied forth & sent out officers in every direction to bring in everything that could bear arms. When the Emperor came up, instead of meeting recruites; met a formidable enemy who surrounded & took him prisoner. He was court marshaled & condemned & shot at Padilla, on the 19th of that month at 6 ock P.M.

This terminated the unbridled ambition of a despot. He was said to be brave & energetic, but could not bear popularity. A friend & acquaintance of mine who went the year before I did happened to be at Soto Marina when he landed & described his person as imposing. When I saw Genl. Gutieres at Monterey, he was getting he told me a salary of $2,700 per annum as a Military officer. He said that during Iturbide's revolution in Mexico that he (Gutieres) was at Washington endeavouring to get Congress to assist them in their struggle for liberty but not for monarchy. Had Iturbide been satisfied with a Presidency, he could have been sustained. But he aspired to highest penicle of power & fame and such to rise no more.

On my entering Monterey, John Finch took Mr. Fletchers sword & sold or pawned it for brandy & consequently was on a spry until he found I was about to start when he sobered up & came forward to beg my pardon. In the meantime I had learned of his conduct through Mr. Adams Servant to whom he had made propositions to join a few soldiers which were stationed there to lay in ambush upon the road and assassinate us, the two servants joining the soldiers & dividing the spoil among them. Mr. Adams svt. Betrayed his confidence & came to me with the facts, I thanked him very kindly saying that I had no confidence in John as an honest or respectable man but that I did not think he was quite so bad as all that, but I should watch him close.

The day we left I ordered the mules brot in and when we came to pack them John was ready to help & steped forward to catch a mule. I said to him that he might stand back that we had no further need of him.

He expressed some surprise when I told him what I had herd. He denied it bravely but I told him that he had forfeited all claim to my confidence & must not show his face on the road as we should know his intentions to be evil & that we should not hesitate at all to shut him down. That was the last interview I had with John. We left Monterey for Cadarita Mar 1/28 where we arrived at sunset. At this place we found an American doctor also an Italian medico & two or three Frenchmen. One of which is prevailed on to wait a day for him to get his horses from the country & accompany us to the coast. He was so importunate that I consented to wait. The Italian Dr. invited me to dine with him the next day & was quite polite.

In the region the Sugar cane is cultivated largely, from which most of the country north & west is supplied with brown sugar. I did not see their facilities for manufacture but judge they were rude and simple. The climate here I should think healthy & quite agreeable.

The Frenchmans mules not coming in, we concluded to go on & let him follow. Messrs Dazot, Duran & Don Pedro overtook us the 2 day. We proceeded on to Camargo, thense to Renosa & on the 10th March arrived at Matamoras situate[d] 40 miles from the sea on the bank of the Rio del Norte.

We proceeded direct to the Customhouse with the larger part of my funds. Consul Smith met me quite cordially & obtained pasturage for my animals 30 miles from town. I started with them alone & encamped with them in open prairie, got to the ranch at 9 next morning, & returned the next day much fatigued.

Matamoros was supposed to contain at this time 8 or 9,000 inhabitants, mostly Spaniards & apparently poor in the general. There was six or eight brick houses owned by foreigners & mostly tenanted as merchantable establishments.

The men in business at this time were Godfrey, Lord, Smith, Cutters, Tanner, Hale, La Font, Dr. Bowers, Divine, Pendergrass & others. Provisions of all kinds were scarce & dear, Board was worth a dollar a day or $2 pr. month.

The house of business, the change of people & language produced a new era in my carear, presenting future hopes & prospects, in quite a facids [facet] of things. Here I found some from diferent parts of the U.S. & especially one from St. Louis Mo. whose brother I had known for several years. This young man to who I allude had gone to that place under the covers of night, yes a fugitive from justice and the might of dire remorse like an incubus weighed upon him. Not a smile upon his visage to break the sullen gloom that hung his brow in sadness. He had been there some months as clerk for Consul Smith. His sobriety had won for him many friends, but of the canker at the heart no one new ought.

He had taken the life of a worthy citizen in cool blood, the cause he could not assign for there was none.

An imaginary wounded reputation was falsely urged in mitigation of the dreadful crime, but gave no calm or quiet to his meditations & every view of the facts wrote condemnations on his wounded conscience. I mentioned the facts of his case, having been apprised through letter from Missouri, but as yet, no one had learned it there. Among his acquaintances he stood high, & when informed of his dilemma, replied that he could not be taken from there. Such are the fruits of a false education, a wounded honor, an inferred insult, could only be repaired by the pistol, or the bowie knife. Concessions were accounted cowardice, and devout acknowledgements, but pucillanimity.

Mr. Strother was the young man who in the heat of blood & ebullition of anger, deliberately made the resolve to walk into court and ask lawyer Couzins to step out a moment, & while C. was closing the door plunged this fatal dagger to his heart. I say this seems deliberate as time & place gave ample room for reflection. But no doubt his purpose was filled & regardless of consequence, yealded to the dreadful infatuation.

But this was not the only scape gallows I found there, a butcher by the name of Cope committed burglarly while I was there. He was late

at the billiard room one night when no doubt he took observations &
after shutting up the house returned and cautiously took but a window
glass & passed his hand inside & opened the door, went in & took out
$800. My host was in his room in the morning before he had risen, &
urged him to get up, & weigh him some beef. He seemed quite dila-
tory, but leisurely got up. While he was dressing my host was walking
the room with a small cane in this hand when all at once it sunk into
the earth, as if the ground was not solid.

This fact suggested to him that he would run his stick down again,
when he thought it came in contact with coin but said nothing at the
time, but soon it was rumoured that such a house had been robbed &
he immediately made known his discoveries. They went to Mr. Copes
room and soon found a part of his deposit. He was immediately taken
into custody & lodged in jail. Notwithstanding guilt stared him on every
side yet he protested his innocence. A verdict of guilty had already been
publicly announced, & it was folly on his part to wheedle friend or foe,
as punishment in some shape was inevitable. The Americans came to the
conclusion to administer justice in their own way. They bribed the jailor
& obtained admission to the prisoner & in the dead of night took him
by the arms & led him forth in the direction of the woods maintaining
profound silence until they came near where he become quite uneasy
& inquired where they were going with him. They made him little or
no answer but urged forward. Things looked more & more portentious
and altho there were no threats, yet everything had a semblance of ret-
ribution. The guilty facts could but stare him in the face, and exclaim
incessantly, "thou art the man." The mental conflict deepened every
moment, as they neared the outrageous "gol gotcha." He could proceed
no farther, & voluntarily called a halt that he might confess all. This
indication was regarded favourably, & procedure was staid a little, that
he might reveal his nefarious deeds to which he had hitherto arrived
himself innocent. They informed him that if he had anything to say
they would hear it & go no further provided an honest confession &
surrender of the stolen funds should be made. He then described his
other place of deposit being in a brickyard defining it[s] precise location.
Two men were thereupon dispatched to visit the depot & return again

& report progress while the rest of the company remained incognito awaiting their return. The money was found & reported, and the prisoner returned to his cell from whense he had been taken to await further trial. My impression now is that he was afterwards released from jail by some of his friends, and allowed to abscond. I think I learned these facts at Orleans from some one that came from there after I did. And especially as I became acquainted (I think through the same source) of an interesting case that occurred after I left. Two young men came to Matamoras ostensibly for the purpose of buying mules for to drive to the States. My impression is that I saw them there, but am not certain. It appears that they were hanging about there some time, when it so happened, that one of them was passing along near where a young man was laying in the shade his arm over his face apparently asleep. But at the same time peaking from under it and watching the movements of the passenger who in passing a log house seemed to look up toard it quite intently. So much so that the sleepers curosity was awakened.

When the stranger had got out of sight, the lounger concluded to go & see if he could discover anything special in front of the log house. In looking up & saw a hole beneath the end of a beam & at once suspected that something might be secreted there. He climed up so as to introduce his hand when it came in contact with a large roll of counterfeit Bills comprising branches of the U.S. Bank.

The young man went immediately to the Consul & reported his discovery. I disremember the amt. found but was several thousand. Arrest was made of them both, & they were conveyed over to Orleans with all the necessary evidences for their conviction, & they were put up on the chain gang as scavengers in the city.

On the 10 Apr I visited the sea shore for the first time in my life, in company with Consul Smith who kindly offered to assist me in carrying aught I had that was "needful" as he rode in a gig having a box under the seat, while I was on horse back. I handed over to him a few hundred Pesos, while I carried as much bullard as I thought prudent having to lodge on the way. At our lodging we carried our bags and threw them under the bed we slept in fearing no danger & no one said why doze? So, morning came & all was right.

After breakfast we pursued our journey to the Brazos, where we found several from Matimoras with whom we were acquainted and also made the acquaintance of several Captains of vessels then laying in port.

Brazos Santiago (arms of St. James) lies directly opposite to point Isabella where the troops were stationed for some time, at the commencement of the war with Mexico. It contained but a few houses at that time, as it stood upon the naked beach entirely destitute of vegetation or comfort. Our time there was a routine of conviviality commingling with Captains of Schooners, sailors, citizens & oistermen, who constituted no unimportant part of our community, as we were furnished with fresh oisters every evening.

I returned to Matamoras, hired a muleteer to take my effects to the Brassas on the 8th Apr. We had to cross the Rio del Norte and also an area of the sea by a ferry boat, swimming the mules. At the last ferry, I opened my trunk, & took out a bag of some $600 also an ingot of gold, & then told the muleteer to stop at the vice Consuls, & leave the trunk & not take it to the Custom house with the cash loads & at the same time throwing my bag across my saddle, mounted & went forward alone; When I had got some miles from the ferry a Spaniard overtook me, & said the muleteer wished to see me. I asked him what he wanted, but he pretended not to know the cause, but said he wanted to see me. I whirled & went back & found him still at the ferry. I asked him what he wanted, he said he could not leave my trunk at the Consuls, but would have to take it to the Custom House. Never mind said I, you take it to the Consuls, & I will see you are satisfied for it. "*Mui bien Señor*" he replied. I left him & went on again alone musing as proceeded upon the consequences of being apprehended & suffering confiscation it being evident that I was in the act of smuggling, and I naturally began to look around on every side for some secret depot where I could lodge the contraband until night & then take it to the consul without risk. But it seemed to be an entire sameness for I could find no special object that I could identify & moreover the caravan was behind me & would be cognizant to the facts & I saw no other alternative but press boldly forward in the midst of the custom house guard who continually patrolling under sworn vigilance, to protect the revinue. Moreover my indecision soon brought me in full view of the village & harbor & all was there descided to go ahead sink or swim. The day was warm & fortunately I had a good screen under which to hide my treasure, in the ample covering of a large Spanish Cloak; with this protection I rrode boldly up to the door of the [U.]S. Consuls where I chanced to see Mr. Green of Matamoras a particular friend & who could sympathize with those who justly, altho illegally were trying to save their just earnings for he had suffered the confiscation of a considerable amt of goods some years previous which he had brought from Baltimore.

As I saw him I called to him to come to me; he came out in a twinkling & the precious charge was soon beyond the reach of vulgar eyes. It was but a few minutes until the *"attajo"* came up and said mules with the trunk was snatched from the herd, with the dexterity of a Spaniard & unladen in a gift & the mule passed on. This took place within a stones jerk of the Custom house & no one said aught pro or con. Hitherto I conceited myself exceedingly fortunate in the game of smuggling, but there still remained further, prestige necessary before it should be beyond the reach of the vigilant eye of the law.

I had engaged my passage with Capt. Parker who agreed to take me & my money for $80 to New Orleans & being conversant with my financial affairs, favoured the transit of my cash from the Consuls iron chest, to some place incognito on shipboard. We were in the habit every evening of buying out the oister men & setting the sailors to roasting while all were made welcome to participate in this discussion. When 9 ock arrived the Capt. would remark "anything to go aboard Dr?" yes *Sir* I replied come upstairs with me, a hint would pass from him to the sailors standing around who without explanation followed us to the Iron safe where each one received 2 rolls of $25 which was balanced in their pea Jacket pockets & then without show of guilt or crime walked boldly on board the vessel. I led the way descending to the cabin adroitly lifting a birth matress & casting our charge beneath it & at the same time remarking to the mate to take notice & act accordingly. He replied in sailor phrase "aye aye Sir" & at the same time observing that he could hide it where he could scarcely find himself.

He had sawed a little 8 by 10 trap window in the back of a birth through which he could run his arm & place things above the sealing of the birth where none would be likely to suspect a contraband depot. After all was deposited I went above where a Sergeant & two soldiers were passing the deck, the former came up to me knowing that I could talk Spanish & said to me that from all that he could discover there was smuggling going on. Aye said I of this you better be quite certain or it might go ill with you for the Captain is a furious fellow & if wrongfully accused will throw your boys overboard. You better be quite certain the captain coming on deck at the same time. I remarked to him that the Sergeant was apprehensive of our smuggling, when he began to swear furiously in English but the officers understood the purport and remained whist.

My bolts of money which came from the custom house were laid on the cabin floor & I would here remark that each bolt contained $1,400 first rolled in canvass & sewed $25 each then placed longitudinally in green oxhide which being soak together & sewed firm with a thong & afterwards dried became as solid as a stick of wood in affect. Two of these bolts made a convenient load for a mule & could be lashed to a pack saddle without much trouble. (*I find from my record, that I smugled in all at the coast some $2,400. I sent down $900 by two young Doctors, then by the consul & myself $1,500 saving in duties $84.) We remained in port several days waiting for deeper water upon the bar. At length two or three vessels being ready to embark started out, first with one & then another having two or three boats crews on deck to assist in passing the bar.

One boat proceeded ours & got safely through & anchored. The hands then came back & having cast a small anchor away forward with a hasser[76] attached to it was then brot on board our deck where the hands began to haul & which they continued until the anchor came home as they term it, & the cry all safe was heard for a moment, but we were soon apprised that we were still in the channel or rather had not passed through it, and great peril was inevitable unless we could keep the channel & work back into harbour. The wind was in the south &

---

[76]A hawser is a large cable for mooring a ship.

blew heavily carrying onto what was called the north breakers & every minute was driving us upon its shoals. & hense every heavy mass would lift us up but on receding rants let us down with a vengeance. For a few moments situation was alarming indeed, fears were entertained that the vessel would spring a leak & fill with water. I was delighted in seeing the sagasity of our cabin boy who apprehending the danger of being blown high & dry availed himself of some small ropes which he tied around my species bolts, that they could be drawn to deck in case of stranding. By dint of effect however the vessel was gotten back to the channel & floated into harbor again.

On the 16th Apr we made another & successful trial & at 6 P.M. found ourselves afloat on the ocean for the first time. Darkness soon closed upon us & I retired to birth, as seasickness immediately effected me. The waves were high, frequently dashing across our deck; the bilge water surged from side to side & while having become stagnant gave off a most nacious stench which was alone sufficient to provoke emesis. I was greatly exercised for two days with ineffectual heavings, & it was only by dint of entire prostration that I could keep secrets or subdue my passions, and what made it more perplexing was some 15 or 20 Spaniards were in the same cabin who could speak no English and I was made the medium of communication between them and the Cabin Boy, and it is not easy to imagine how numerous the wants of such persons are, laboring under continual excessive qualm.

But we were nearing my native land, & the friends I held dear, from whom I had been separated eleven years. At the end of two days the gale subsided & I was enabled to get one deck once more in a reduced state of health, but on the heels of convalescence.

On the 21st the Captain took observations at 12 & found our latitude to be 28–27 ms and our distance one hundred & thirty miles from the Billies[77] which hove in sight at daylight next morning. Towards noon we descried the Pilot approaching us who took the helm & stove to

---

[77]Fort de La Belize, in Louisiana, was a French fort and settlement built and inhabited in 1699 near the mouth of the Mississippi River. In 1721 the first lighthouse-type structure, rising 62 feet, was constructed at that location. It was one of the first permanent settlements inside the current boundaries of the state of Louisiana. David Roth, *Louisiana Hurricane History* (Camp Springs, Md.: National Weather Service), 12, http://www.wpc.ncep.noaa.gov/research/lahur .pdf (accessed August 1, 2014).

make the S.W. Pass but without success the wind being directly a head. We beat about for some hours but finding it utterly useless, cast anchor.

Dinner was brought upon deck & served up most ludicrous by having to eat with our hand & hold our plates with the other or all was overboard. Having scraped a little acquaintance with the Pilot he proposed that the Capt. & myself should accompany him on shore. I readily acceded to the proposition & soon I found myself upon terrafirma again.

The Pilot was occupying a comfortable cottage on the river bank which at that place [was] quite a narrow peninsular of land made by successive accumulations of floating sand brought down by the father of rivers. O it was good to sit down again in a state of quiet after having been tossed for six days in vile endurance, but the transition was the more elating as it was sudden & radical. We had availed ourselves of fresh water some 3 or 4 ms. out at sea having entered the channel of the river which had not yet commingled with the briny deep but as if conscious of its own puragatives, maintained its proud course into the bosom of the world of yealding waters.

The Captain & Pilot after a little refreshment returned to the vessel to spend the night, or at the first favourable breeze were through the pass into the river. I was kindly invited to remain with the Pilots family until they should get into the river.

We had *sin ceremonia* [without ceremony] a fine supper of oisters with some vegetables & all smacked savorily my appetite having become keen and craving. The family retired early & to me perhaps sleep was never sweeter than on that memorable night. The world with all its charms & all its ills lay in sweet oblivion until at daylight I was brought into a state of sensibility by the strange sound of the tow boat. Porpus or Porssus, which went puffing by in search of vessels that could not assend the river unaided. It soon returned with a Brig on one side & a Schooner on the other.

About 8 ock our Schooner came sailing up but instead of stopping for me glided silently by. I greatly wondered the Captain should forget me, or that he should pass me unherded, fearing that the former was the case, I hired a man to take me in a skiff & persue the Scooner which it appeared had passed up to a customhouse where it lay too until I arrived. When I got on board I looked at my hands & to my surprise counted ten blisters, but I was on board & all was well.

The Officer came to me & asked me if I had any contraband. I replied that I was not aware that I had but he could serch my trunk if thought best when he replied that he was satisfied without serch. Business being concluded, we were soon under way & the wind being fresh we got to Fort Jackson at dusk, where we laid too the wind having laid, but at eleven it improved again, & we spread sail, but made but little progress until morning when it blew almost a gale. When we came to the English bend at 3 P.M. We found several vessels lying at anchor not daring to risk a trial as the bend in the river brought the wind almost directly ahead.

Our mate however was a brave seaman & proposed to the Capt. to put on what he termed the "bonnet" and in so doing he was confident that we could weather the point without hazard. The Capt. acceeded to his proposition & we returned, but not without evident intimidation as we would frequently be on the cress but would right again as the gust would pass over.

The Spaniards became quite alarmed on seeing the evident signs of danger & especially thinking the Capt. apprehensive. It was some hours before we got past the bend but at length succeeded.

We arrived at Orleans at Six, having been 31 hours from the Bellise, distance one hundred & fifteen miles.

On board our vessel, were a number of Spaniards, & one of them to all appearance, in a state of indigene [indigence]. The captain said it was doubtful whether the municipality would (not) prevent his landing him, unless he was better clad, & it was understood by a few of us that we would do something for him before he landed. I accordingly striped off my entire suit & presented it to the old man, which he denied in good earnest.

The cabin boy was also entitled to some nummeration in addition to my kind regards for his cheerful attentions, not only to my own wants, but to those who through my aquntcy [acquaintancy] had participated in his services.

The next day I took boarding at $5 per week & dragged my specie to the U.S. Branch Bank where I exchanged it for paper at par. The teller gave it to me mostly in $1.00 bills. I looked at it a moment & said to myself has my all dwindled down to this little measure? We had trogd [trudged] in landing and unlanding the little packs for better than three months and it had been the darling of my care all the way from Chihuahua to Matamoras a distance of 800 miles, & then 800 by sea, but now my mind was lifted above the sordid dust & it now smugly ensconced within the iron valts of Uncle Sams Bank, while its representative was as smugly encinctured upon my person.

New Orleans was quite a business place then, some 200 sail were laying too besides a large number of steam and flat boats. I soon engaged my passage to St. Louis on the St. Boat *Courtland*, Captain Agerton[78] master.[79]

During my stay of three or four days I passed through the city generally visiting the cemetary which I was shocked to find so dilapidated & abused. There were many fine monuments, originally, but dreadfully effaced & mutilated.

Our boat was freighted with United States troops bound for Greenbay.[80] The officers were Col. Taylor (since President),[81] Capt. Smith, Leiut. Juett, Leiut. McKinsey, Leiut. Reynolds, & Leiut. Jarey together with one hundred & forty five Soldiers. The young officers I found quite social & orderly. Col. T appeared to be an unassuming modest man, not overly talkative, but sufficiently so to be agreeably entertaining. I little thought that the highest honor of the nation then awaited him, but he was in the line of preferment and ten or fifteen years often makes great changes in human affairs, and the exaltation of men seems often fortuitous, and not infrequently the result of sequential routine favouring the destined achme.

---

[78]Captain Edgerton operated the steamboat *Cortland*.

[79]An amendment to the Steamboat Act of 1838 made it unlawful for anyone who had not served in some capacity for three years to take command as master of a steamboat. Not until the Steamboat Act of 1871 was a steamboat captain required to have a license. Hunter and Hunter, *Steamboats on the Western Rivers*, 237.

[80]The soldiers were most likely traveling to Fort Howard, a military fort first built in 1816.

[81]Zachary Taylor was a career officer in the U.S. Army before becoming the twelfth president of the United States in March 1849.

Having mentioned the names of the officers above, or becoming acquainted with them more or less, felt an interest in their welfare thereafter, and hense I think it proper to mention a circumstance attending the fate of Leiut. McKinsey one of the most amiable of them all & beloved by every body. I think it was 1829 that he fell substitutionally a victim to dire revenge. It seems that a soldier had a pique against a corporal for some imaginary insult, & deliberately made up his mind to take his life under semblance of duty. This soldier being on guard one night & supposing his adversary was the corporal of the guard, concluded to hail his approach & irrespective of counter sign shoot him down. But who should the corporal of the guard be but the beloved McKinsey who fell dead at his feet. His death was greatly lamented by all who knew him.[82]

Nothing special transpired on our way up to impede our progress, all was comfort & harmony. We arrived at the Barracs[83] six ms below St. Louis where we called for an hour & visited the several building[s] then being erected. Their Hospital of brick was nearly completed. The rest of the buildings were mostly of stone. Col. Taylor was received by the officers in garrison with marked attention, while he returned dignified salutation. We were all soon on board again & proceeded to St. Louis where we arrived at 1 ock P.M. We had not been in port before I had the pleasure to meet my old Preceptor & several other acquaintances. It having been reported through the Santa fee trains, that the young Dr. was signally fortunate in practice & had accumulated a "heap" rendered my enterance into the city cordial at least.

---

[82]On September 8, 1828, Lieutenant John Mackenzie was the officer in charge at Fort Crawford the evening one of the more highly regarded and educated soldiers drank too much, then shot and killed Lt. Mackenzie. Another solider witnessed Lt. Mackenzie "calling to the corporal of the guard, and told him to 'take that fellow to the guard-house.' Hardly had the order escaped his lips, when Reneka observed him, and instantly poising his rifle, shot Mackenzie through the brain. It was a long shot, but a deadly one. In making it, Reneka had killed his bosom friend. He was arrested and confined in the guard-house, and when he became sane, and learned he had killed his best friend, no words of mine can picture the heart-rending agony of remorse that seized him. But he was delivered over to the civil authorities, convicted of murder, and sentenced to be hung and brought back here to be executed." Consul Willshire Butterfield, *History of Crawford and Richland Counties, Wisconsin* (Springfield, Ill.: Union Publishing Co., 1884), 329–54.

[83]Jefferson Barracks, a U.S. Army post started in 1826.

I made several visits through the day & at evening I was invited together with several gentlemen by Capt. Edgerton to spend the evening in his cabin to quaff a few bottles of wine & participate in a game of whist[84] for pass time only.

The next day I took passage to St. Charles from which place I had started three years before & where I had spent eight years of my life, four as a mechanic, three in study and one in practice. Here also I found the monument of my mechanical enterprise, & which three years before comprised my all. It was but a small talent, but by dint of constant perseverance in well doing, & had more than doubled its value. During my studentship, it paid me three hundred pr. annum, & safely carried me through, besides an out fit for my southern tour. But it was now worth less than when I left it, as its rents were greatly reduced. It had been nevertheless a kind of handmaid to a better fortune. Through its income I have acquired my hitherto modest eminance.

Having begun with nothing, I could now wield the original, together with some $6,500 in addition. This apparent fortuity was self consoling, & I confess sometimes elevating to my mind, but I think I never lost the balance of equanimity & self control. As to medical acquirement, I felt wanting; altho I had been as I thought a good student, but I still needed a better polish, & other opportunities that I could not get in the far west at that time. But suffice it to say, that eight years had wrought a great change in my circumstances, it seemed to me almost unsought for, tho modesty desired. The course that led to my good fortune, was altogether unpremeditated; a bare livelihood was anticipated but nothing extra of fortunes partiality did I even crave, above my competitors.

At St. Charles I found signal changes had taken place among the inhabitants. Some had removed to other countries, & some to that bourn from which none ever return. What old acquaintances I found met me cordially. Even Dr. Wilson who while I was a student seemed rather to look upon me in the light of competitor if not usurper, could now greet me with the utmost cordiality, and even seemed to

---

[84]The classic game of whist is a plain-trick card game for four players (two teams of partners), using a full deck. It was played widely in the eighteenth and nineteenth centuries.

recognized equality. As they say in that country "I did not let on" but all passed off admirably.

I immediately went out to Dr. Millingtons farm a little in the rear of town, where I found him cultivating largely the Palma Christi & manufacturing extensively the Oil vicini. He also had dabbled largely in horticulture, & every way full of enterprize. He was the elder Bro. of my Preceptor, who had declined practice soon after his brothers arrival, throwing it into his hands.

I returned to St. Louis in a day or two where I engaged my passage on board the Steamboat *Maryland* Capt. Lindle master price $15. We arrived at Louisville in a little less than four days. At Shippingsport we took a hack & went up to Louisville & in company with Cpt. Lindle visited the principal port of the city [and] found it a place of considerable community.

At C[incinnati] I found some old acquaintances and among them was Timothy Flint[85] who I had often heard preach at St. Charles, Missouri he having been sent out by the Presbiterian Missionary board in the year 1816. He was now editing a phamplet stated the *"Western Review."* He was glad to see me & was importunate that I should furnish him with a sketch of my Mexican travels. I allowed him to extract from my diary an article of considerable lenth & also furnished him with a succinct account of the Mexican people & country, which he after publishing in his "Review" republished in a Book of Adventures written by himself from notes furnished by a young man by the name of James Patty comprising a tour through New Mexico & its western

---

[85]Timothy Flint (1780–1840) was born in North Reading, Massachusetts. After graduation from Harvard College in 1800, Flint went on to study theology for two years and was ordained pastor of the church in Lunenburg, Massachusetts. In 1814 he resigned his pastorate and began missionary work in New England, eventually moving west and settling in Cincinnati. A year later Flint and his family moved to Saint Louis and then to Saint Charles for two years, where Willard heard Flint preach. In 1826 Flint published a memoir of his adventures throughout the Mississippi River Valley titled *Recollections of the Last Ten Years Passed in the Valley of the Mississippi*. In 1827 he started working at the *Western Monthly Review* as an apprentice writer and by 1830 was the editor. From 1827 to 1833 he also wrote two travel books and four novels. In Flint's later years his failing health caused him to return to New England. He spent the remainder of his days in North Reading, where he passed away on August 18, 1840. Folsom, *Timothy Flint*, 13–73.

miles reaching to the Californias with thrilling incidents pertaining to the imprisionment of the party & there ultimate release, & particularly the death of his father in prision before releasement.

The narrative was the more interesting to me, in as much as I was well acquainted with his father off & on from the year 1817 to some year prior to his death which occurred I think in [18]29. His last expedition was concocted at my office in [18]27 he with several others having visited Chihuahua to release the Copper mines of Mr. Guerra of which I may have made mention before. But as they could not agree on the term of compensation Mr. Patty & his partners concluded to get up the trapping expedition that resulted in the calamities they experienced in California & set forth in his narration.

Parson Flint had laid asside his clerical robes & taken the editorial chair, which purhapse was a more efficient means of subsistence, & I apprehend for more congenial to his didactic principles.

The leadings of his genius showed a proclivity to romance & novel, & needed but a skeleton of fact to make a protracted story. His *"Francis Beaning"* and *"Backwoodsman"*[86] were specimens, and being of a rather bilious temperaments, indulged in acetic recrimination amounting to constitution at petulance.

His notice of my Mexican sojourn being twice published tended to place me in rather more than ordinary prominence. Among my young compears & especially as Mexico at that time was as foreign as the antipode, commerce & communications not yet having been established.

News from Palestine now is far more frequent than Mexican news at that time. Commercial negotiations by land & sea were just beginning to develop & American adventurers had found way into a few of their seaports but mostly by a land route to Sta. Fee in New Mexico.

But the U.S. were nearly as ignorant of them as they were of us but few of them had ever been further than Orleans north & consequently as isolated from us, as if separated by a Chinese Wall. But the war

---

[86]Dr. Willard is referring to Timothy Flint's *Francis Berrian, or the Mexican Patriot*, first published in Boston in 1826, and *George Mason, the Young Backwoodsman: or, "Don't Give Up the Ship." A Story of the Mississippi*, published in Boston in 1829. Ibid., 14.

of old Spain having ended, & a simi Republican government having been adopted, the door of enterprise was opened, & a rapid ingress of Adventurers was the result.

It was often remarked by Americans who had been in Mexico so that such men the facinations of the climate, & novelty of the people, that a return to that country was nearly always desirable. Tis true, much can be said in its favour, & many things to its disparagement; and all things considered, it may be a question perhaps, whether our section of the globe is more redundant of natural blessing than another. With the exception of the frigid or archtic regions where all things are considered, it might be hard to make choice a Mexican temperature considered on the scheme of comfort would be descidedly preferable, but withstanding the congeniality of temperature an eternal aridity prevails, & little or nothing releases the monotony of the landscape, but a chance shrub, or annoying thorns & thistly or an occasional palm tree or aloe plant indigenous to the country can be seen.

No such aspect of flowing forest clad in verdant sheen, to cheer the many traveler & screen him from the mid day sun, as abound in our temperate grasses & mark the revolving seasons, & make up our sensibilities to cold, & heat, & to the imperitive necessity of laying up in summer for the approaching winter.

In the fall of [18]29 as the symptoms of winter commenced, I came to the conclusion to migrate to a warm climate & consequently in company with some fifteen Spaniards who through my influence embarked with me on board of Steam boat *Sampson*, Capt. Wallace offering to reduce my passage I think ten dollars in consequence.

We had quite a pleasant time on the trip having the confidence of Capt. & his Spanish guests & often called upon as interpreter on the way.

Arriving at Orleans Dec. 2, 1829, I met with my old messmate Mr. Marble who was keeping a public house on Benville Street[87] in Company with Mr. Parkerson lately from Natchez. I gladly took boarding with them at $7 per week.

---

[87]This public house was on Bienville Street in the French Quarter of New Orleans, Louisiana.

At this place I also found several old acquaintances from St. Louis who together with other associates which I soon found made my sojourn then quite pleasant indeed. I remained I think until some time in February where I embarked for Mobile Alabama. During my stay at Orleans I spent most of my time in reading & writing, sometimes enjoying myself rambling over the city and its suburbs.

I was often gratified with meeting old acquaintances from St. Louis, Cincinnati & other places & among the rest was Col Ward my old fellow traveler from Sta Fee to Carasal in Mexico, he was now on his return to that country having been appointed by Congress Consul to some point I think Durango. He seemed greatly pleased to see me, and offered me an equal interest with him in any speculations we might make, & participation in the involvements of his consulship. But I thought it not best, & pacified him with the assurance that my funds were all or nearly so in Cincinnati which would make it necessary for me to return there soon. We had a series of pleasant pass time while he remained, and on one occasion he invited Mr. Marble, Douglass, Moorehouse, D. Johnson, Capt. Lee & myself to an oister supper at Browns Hotel where we spent the evening.

Col. Paul Anderson was part owner of the Steam boat *Uncle Sam*. We had other social spirits among whom Col. Anderson was not the least, nor was he destitute of a good degree of chivalrous gallantry peculiar to the batchelors of his age for he must have verged upon fifty. So far as I could read him, he was temperate in all things except laquacity.

But it was quite different with his brother Bill with whom I became acquainted in New Mexico, he was also a batchelor, but a confirmed drinker yet seldom found drunk. He possessed a good degree of human kindness & laid me under a tribute of respect, for his marked regard for me, when first a stranger in the country. If he ever had received any domestic polish, the sacrifices had become so marred & effaced, by grog bruising, that he aspired to little or no intellectual [ease man] but chose rather to heard among the lower tribes of bipeds. I could but appreciate however his warmth of friendship & repeated kindness during my stay in New Mexico.

Dr. Willard's Medical Books

PHYSICIANS, STUDENTS, AND general readers may be interested to learn which medical books guided Dr. Willard in his medical apprenticeship. Fortunately, in his autobiography Dr. Willard provided a list of the authors and medical subjects he studied. Rowland Willard studied primarily under Dr. Jeremiah Millington, who attended the first medical school established in the United States, at the University of Pennsylvania in Philadelphia, along with his brother, Seth Millington. The subjects listed in Willard's medical books followed the curriculum presented by the medical school where both Millington brothers graduated. In the fall of 1828 Dr. Willard enrolled as a student at Jefferson College in Philadelphia to continue his medical education for a few months.

William Barton was a surgeon of the Naval Hospital at Philadelphia and a professor of botany at the University of Pennsylvania. His book, *Vegetable Material Medica of the United States or Medical Botany* (Philadelphia: M. Carey & Son, 1817–18), is filled with colored engravings. As a botanist Dr. Barton recognized that Lewis and Clark's early nineteenth-century government-sponsored explorations of the western United States introduced the medical community to dietetic plants utilized by the indigenous people. In the second edition of the book, Dr. Barton acknowledges the scientific contributions of Baron Alexander von Humboldt from his travels in Mexico prior to returning to Paris in 1804.

Charles Bell was a surgeon at the hospital of Edinburgh. He wrote his book, *A System of Operative Surgery: Founded on the Basis of Anatomy* (London: Longman, Hurst, Rees & Orme, 1807–1809), based on his practical experience. His work is original in that he provided descriptions of the surgeries he performed. He relied heavily on his strict education in anatomy and benefited greatly from assisting and partnering with his brother, John Bell. In his writing Charles Bell encouraged critical thinking by attempting to train the medical student in deductive reasoning as to probable occurrences.

John Bell provided descriptions of diseases and operations in his book *The Principles of Surgery* (New York: Collins & Perkins, 1810). In the second edition, J. Augustine Smith abridged Dr. Bell's work. The book addresses hemorrhages, fractures of all sorts, and obstructions and tumors throughout the body.

James Hamilton was a senior physician to the Royal Infirmary and other hospitals of Edinburgh for thirty years prior to the publication of his book, *Observation of the Utility and Administration of Purgative Medicines in Several Diseases with Additional Observations and Cases* (Edinburgh: Constable, 1811). Hamilton was also a corresponding member of the Medical Lyceum of Philadelphia. He advocated purging the body using purgative medicines in order to restore a patient's appetite and improve digestion. It was a delicate balance between obviating constipation and at the same time avoiding full purging.

Samuel Merriman was a medical doctor affiliated with the Royal Academy of Science at Siena. Dr. Merriman studied hundreds of pregnant women and monitored difficult births. After studying 150 women, he determined that the average pregnancy lasted thirty-nine weeks. He recorded his results in his book, *A Synopsis of the Various Kinds of Difficult Parturition: with Practical Remarks on the Management of Labor* (Philadelphia: Thomas Dobson, 1816).

Joseph Priestley's *History and Present State of Discoveries Relating to Vision, Light and Colours* (London: J. Johnson, 1772) was one of the earliest works on optics and the most comprehensive of its time. Published in just one English edition, it remained the only English work on the subject for 150 years. To Americans, Priestley was better known as a defender of the colonies' right to freedom. Willard also read Priestley's *Familiar Introduction to the Theory and Practice of Perspective* (London: J. Johnson, 1780).

A. Philips Wilson was a medical doctor and admitted as a fellow of the Royal College of Physicians in Edinburgh in 1795. Later, he became a fellow at the Royal College of Physicians in London and the Royal Society while operating a large and successful practice in London. His *Treatise on Febrile Diseases* (Hartford, Conn.: Oliver D. Cooke, 1809) represents his most comprehensive research volume and was translated into both German and French. Wilson thought that inflammation such as vomiting and coughing resulted from the body's attempt to remove whatever was causing it not to function properly.

Caspar Wistar was a medical doctor and professor of anatomy at the University of Pennsylvania. His book, *A System of Anatomy for the Use of Students of Medicine* (Philadelphia: T. Dobson & Son, 1817), was originally designed as a text for anatomy lecture courses at the university, as well as for the benefit of practitioners. Dr. Wistar wrote about the structure of bones and cartilage and how bone is formed. His text discusses all parts of the body from the head to the trunk, including superior and interior extremities as well as the muscular system.

Dr. Willard's Accounts, 1828

THE FOLLOWING EXCERPT from Dr. Willard's personal accounting pertains to his liquidation of his assets in Chihuahua in 1828. The accounts reveal the cost of his trip to the United States including servant wages, pasturage for the animals, and duties on his cash. Road expenses included meals and lodging and miscellaneous purchases and bribes. Upon his arrival in New Orleans he purchased American clothes and a steamboat ticket. Upon arrival in St. Charles he either purchased medicines from Dr. Millington or paid off this account for medicines received in Chihuahua. He returned to New York to visit his parents and other family members. While there he paid the mortgage on his parents' land. The last account reflects his expenses incurred when he attended classes at Jefferson Medical College in Philadelphia.

Dt	Cash		Contra		Cr	1
1828			1828			
Jan. 22	To Spanish Mill Dollars	$7,161.00	Jan. 22	By loss on Mineral speculation	$450.00	
Apr. 22	,, Sales of 5 mules & 2 horses	175.00	"	,, Duties on money in part 2 per ct.	80.00	
	,, Saddles &c.	24.00	"	,, Power of Attorney	11.00	
	,, Sundries	17.00	30	,, Supposed amt. Horses & Mules	300.00	
			"	,, Servants hire to the coast	33.00	
			Feb. 26	,, Duties on cash	35.00	
			March 10	,, Road expenses to coast	70.00	
			31	,, Board at Matamoras	21.25	
			"	,, Pasturage	7.00	
			Apr 12	,, Transportation to Brazas	10.00	
			"	,, Goods or merchandise	6.00	
			"	,, Sundries	6.84	
			16	,, 3 1/2 pr. Cent Duties on Cash	122.50	
			25	,, Passage to Orleans pr ct on Cash	80.00	
		7,377.00	14	By Balance in Bank	6,144.41	
					7,377.00	

Dt	Cash		Contra	Cr	2
1828		1828			
May 1st	To Balance from Cr side	$6,144.00	Apl. 26	By Merchandise (Raiment)	$45.25
			May 11	,, SteamBoat Passage from N Orleans to St. Louis Mo.	30.00
			19	,, Sundries at do	6.00
			23	,, Passage to Louisville	15.00
			"	,, J.M. Millington a/c	60.50
			25	,, Passage to Cincinnati	5.00
			26	,, do to Cleveland by St	14.00
			Jan. 1	,, Passage & other expenses to Williamson [NY]	25.87½
			July 7	,, Presents to Family	53.00
			"	,, Deed for Land in Williamson	400.00
			Sept 2	,, Passage & other expenses to Vermont	28.50
			Oct. 4	,, Sundries	22.37½
			16	,, Passage &c to N. York	29.71
				,, do to Philadelphia	5.25
		6,144.00		,, By Balance in Bank	5,403.95
					6,144.4

Dt	Cash		Contra		Cr 3
1828			1828		
Oct. 16	To Balance from Cr. Side	$5,403.95	Oct. 17	By Dress Coat	$30.00
				,, Sundry small clothing &c.	15.75
				,, Passage &c to N York & back again	12.87½
			Nov. 12	,, College & Alums house Tickets	116.50
				,, Books and Papers	17.00
				,, Boarding	16.75
				,, Room wood & candles	6.18¾
				,, Sundries (raiment &c)	28.64
			1829	,, Surgical Instruments	7.75
			Mar. 18	,, Passenger to Baltimore &c.	8.00
				,, Do To Wheeling & other a/c	20.00
				,, ,, To Cincinnati	12.00
			14	By Balance in Bank	5,068.00
		5,403.95			5,403.95

Bibliography

All Trails Lead to Santa Fe: An Anthology Commemorating the 400th Anniversary of the Founding of Santa Fe, New Mexico, in 1610. Foreword by Marc Simmons. Preface by Orlando Romero. Santa Fe: Sunstone Press, 2010.

Almada, Francisco R. *Diccionario de Historía, Geografía y Biografía Chihuahuenses.* 2nd ed. Ciudad Juárez: Impresora de Juárez, 1968.

———. *Gobernadores del Estado de Chihuahua.* Chihuahua: Centro Librero la Prensa, 1980.

Alonzo, Armondo. *Tejano Legacy: Rancheros and Settlers in South Texas, 1734–1900.* Albuquerque: University of New Mexico Press, 1998.

Barry, Louise. *The Beginning of the West.* Topeka: Kansas State Historical Society, 1972.

Bell, John R. *The Journal of Captain John R. Bell: The Official Journalist of the Stephen H. Long Expedition to the Rocky Mountains, 1820.* Edited by Harlan Fuller and Leroy R. Hafen, Vol. 6 of *The Far West and the Rockies.* Glendale, Calif.: A. H. Clark, 1954–61.

Benson, Maxine. *From Pittsburgh to the Rocky Mountains: Major Stephen Long's Expedition, 1819–1820.* Golden, Colo.: Fulcrum, 1998.

Benson, Nettie Lee. *The Provincial Deputation in Mexico: Harbinger of Provincial Autonomy, Independence, and Federalism.* Austin: University of Texas Press, 1992.

Blackmar, F. *Kansas: A Cyclopedia of State History.* Vol. 2. Chicago: Standard Publishing, 1912.

Boyle, Susan Calafate. *Los Capitalistas: Hispano Merchants and the Santa Fe Trade.* Albuquerque: University of New Mexico Press, 1997.

Brown, William E. *The Santa Fe Trail: The National Park Service 1963 Historic Site Survey.* St. Louis: Patrice Press, 1988.

Bryan, William Smith, and Robert Rose. *A History of the Pioneer Families of Missouri.* St. Louis: Bryan Brand and Co., 1876.

Cady, A. Howard. *Loto: A Brief History of the Origin of the Game with a Few Notes and Anecdotes in Connection with It and a Description of How to Play It.* New York: American Sports Publishing, 1896.

Chavez, Fray Angelico. *But Time and Chance: The Story of Padre Martinez of Taos, 1793–1867.* Santa Fe: Sunstone, 1981.

Clapsaddle, David. "Mexican Money/American Commerce." *Wagon Tracks* 28, no. 4 (2014): 1–32.

Cosio, Rosa Maria Meyer, and Delia Anaya, eds. *Los inmigrantes en el mundo de los negocios, siglos XIX y XX.* Mexico: INAH, 2003.

Coues, Elliot, ed. *The Expeditions of Zebulon Montgomery Pike.* New York: F. P. Harper, 1895.

Dary, David. *The Santa Fe Trail: Its History, Legends, and Lore.* New York: Penguin, 2000.

———. *Frontier Medicine.* New York: Knopf, 2008.

Dunglison, Robley, M.D., LL.D. *Medical Lexicon: A Dictionary of Medical Science.* Philadelphia: Henry C. Lea, 1874.

Field, Matthew C. *Matt Field on the Santa Fe Trail.* Collected by Clyde and Mae Reed Porter. Edited by John E. Sunder. Norman: University of Oklahoma Press, 1960.

Folsom, James K. *Timothy Flint.* New York: Twayne, 1965.

Franzwa, Gregory M. *Maps of the Santa Fe Trail.* St. Louis: Patrice Press, 1989.

Goodspeed Publishing Company. *History of Adair, Sullivan, Putnam & Schuyler Counties, Missouri.* Vol. 2. Chicago: Goodspeed Publishing Co., 1888.

Gove, Philip Babcock, ed. *Webster's Third New International Dictionary.* Springfield, Mass.: Merriam-Webster, 1986.

Graf, Leroy P. *Economic History of the Lower Rio Grande Valley, 1820–1875.* London: Cambridge University Press, 1942.

Gregg, Josiah. *Commerce of the Prairies.* Norman: University of Oklahoma Press, 1954.

Gregg, Kate. *The Road to Santa Fe: The Journal and Diaries of George Champlin Sibley and Others Pertaining to the Surveying and Marking of a Road from the Missouri Frontier to the Settlements of New Mexico, 1825–1827.* Albuquerque: University of New Mexico Press, 1952.

Hardy, Robert William Hale. *Travels in the Interior of Mexico, in 1825, 1826, 1827 and 1828.* Glorieta, N.M.: Rio Grande Press, 1977.

Hawk, Charles C. "Camino Antiguos: Trails into the Taos Valley." In Corina Santistevan and Julia Moore, eds., *Taos: A Topical History.* Albuquerque: Museum of New Mexico Press, 2013.

Hendricks, Rick. "Father Manuel Rada, Priest and Advocate for New Mexico, 1821–1843." *Catholic Southwest* 17 (2006): 9–33.

Hernández Sáenz, Luz María. *Learning to Heal: The Medical Profession in Colonial Mexico, 1767–1831.* New York: Peter Lang, 1997.

Hollrah, Paul R. *History of St. Charles County, Missouri (1765–1885)*. Missouri, n.p., 1997.

Hopkins, James F., ed. *Papers of Henry Clay*. Vol. 4, *Secretary of State, 1825–1829*. Lexington: University of Kentucky Press, 1972.

Hordes, Stanley. "The History of the Santa Fe Plaza, 1610–1720." In *All Trails Lead to Santa Fe*, pp. 129–46. Santa Fe: Sunstone Press, 2010.

Houck, Louis. *A History of Missouri, from the Earliest Explorations and Settlements until the Admission of the State into the Union*. Vol. 3. Chicago: R. R. Donnelly and Sons, 1908.

Hunter, Louis O., and Beatrice Jones Hunter. *Steamboats on the Western Rivers: An Economic and Technological History*. Mineola, N.Y.: Dover, 1993.

Jackson, Hal. *Boone's Lick Road: A Brief History and Guide to a Missouri Treasure*. Woodston, Kans.: Trails Press, 2012.

———. *Following the Royal Road*. Albuquerque: University of New Mexico Press, 2006.

Lamar, Howard. *The New Encyclopedia of the American West*. New Haven, Conn.: Yale University Press, 1998.

Lavender, David. *Bent's Fort*. New York: Doubleday, 1954.

Lawson, Rich. "Arrow Rock Ferry Now on the National Register of Historic Places." *Wagon Tracks* 27 (2013): 1–28.

Lundwall, Helen. *Copper Mining in Santa Rita, New Mexico, 1801–1838*. Santa Fe: Sunstone Press, 2012.

Manfred, Frederick. *Lord Grizzly*. Lincoln: University of Nebraska Press, 1983.

Martin, Cheryl English. *Governance and Society in Colonial Mexico: Chihuahua in the Eighteenth Century*. Stanford, Calif.: Stanford University Press, 1996.

Mason, F. "Association Intelligence: A Case of Fungus Humatodes of the Eyeball." *British Medical Journal* 1, no. 214 (1865): 126.

Miller, Michael. "Land, Violence and Death: The Bartolome Baca Grant." New Mexico Office of the State Historian, http://dev.newmexicohistory.org/filedetails.php?fileID=24449 (accessed July 13, 2014).

Missouri Historical Company. *History of Saline County Missouri*. St. Louis: Missouri Historical Co., 1883.

Minge, Alan Ward, ed. and trans. "The Last Will and Testament of Don Severino Martinez." *New Mexico Quarterly* 33 (Spring 1963): 33–56.

Moorhead, Max L. *New Mexico's Royal Road: Trade and Travel on the Chihuahua Trail*. Norman: University of Oklahoma Press, 1958.

Morgan, Phyllis. "Mirages on the Santa Fe Trail." *Wagon Tracks* 24, no. 4 (2010): 1–28.

National Historical Company. *History of Howard and Cooper Counties, Missouri*. St. Louis: National Historical Company, 1883.

Neilson, William. *Webster's New International Dictionary*. Springfield, Mass.: G & C Merriam, 1951.

Oliva, Leo. "The 1829 Escorts." In Leo Oliva, ed., *Confrontation on the Santa Fe Trail*. Woodston, Kans.: Santa Fe Trail Association, 1996.

Orozco, Victor. *El Estado de Chihuahua en el parto de la nación, 1810–1831*. Mexico: El Colegio de Chihuahua, 2007.

Rangel, Antonio. "Vascos en Chihuahua." http://vascosmexico.com/index. php?option=com_content&task=view&id=309&Itemid=43 (last modified September 3, 2010).

Reilly Jr., John. "A Dictionary of Numismatic Names, Their Official and Popular Designations." *American Journal of Numismatics* 50 (1917): 209.

Reséndez, Andrés. "Getting Cured and Getting Drunk: State versus Market in Texas and New Mexico, 1800–1850." *Journal of the Early American Republic* 22 (Spring 2002): 77–103.

Rondé, Philippe. "Voyage dans l'état de Chihuahua (Mexique) 1849–1852." *Le Tour de Monde* (1861): 128–60.

Rothstein, William G. *American Physicians in the Nineteenth Century: From Sects to Science*. London: John Hopkins University Press, 1992.

Senator, Hermann, and M. Litten. *Diseases of the Kidneys and of the Spleen*. Edited by James Herrick. Philadelphia: W. B. Saunders, 1905.

Sims, Harold Dana. *The Expulsion of Mexico's Spaniards, 1821–1836*. Pittsburgh: University of Pittsburgh Press, 1990.

Simmons, Marc. *Spanish Government in New Mexico*. Albuquerque: University of New Mexico Press, 1968.

Simmons, Marc, and Hal Jackson. *Following the Santa Fe Trail: A Guide for Modern Travelers*. Santa Fe: Ancient City Press, 2001.

Sisneros, Samuel. "'She Was Our Mother': New Mexico's Change of National Sovereignty and Juan Bautista Vigil y Alarid, the Last Mexican Governor of New Mexico." In *All Trails Lead to Santa Fe*, pp. 279–300. Santa Fe: Sunstone Press, 2010.

Slusher, Roger. "Lexington and the Santa Fe Trail." *Wagon Tracks* 5, no. 4 (1991): 6–9.

Smith, Ralph Allen. *Borderlander: The Life of James Kirker, 1793–1852*. Norman: University of Oklahoma Press, 1999.

Smith II, Walter B. *America's Diplomats and Consuls of 1776–1865*. Occasional Paper No. 2. Washington, D.C.: Government Printing Office, 1986.

Stanford, John Frederick. *The Stanford Dictionary of Anglicised Words and Phrases*. London: Cambridge University Press, 1892.

Stanley, Charles F. *Life Principle Bible*. Nashville: Thomas Nelson, 2009.

Steele, Volney. *Bleed, Blister, and Purge*. Missoula, Mont.: Mountain Press, 2005.

Stewart, Dave, and Ray Knox. *The Earthquake America Forgot: 2,000 Temblors in Five Months—and It Will Happen Again*. Marble Hill, Mo.: Gutenberg-Richter, 1995, 2005.

Stillman, Chauncey Devereux. *Charles Stillman, 1810–1875.* New York: N.p., 1856.

Sturtevant, William, Alfonso Ortiz, and Charles Lange, eds. *Handbook of North American Indians Southwest.* Vol. 9. Washington: Government Printing Office, 1979.

Torres, Jaime F. *Return to Aztlan: A Journey into an Ancestral Past.* Bloomington, Ind.: Xlibris, 2002.

Thwaites, Reuben Gold. *Early Western Travels, 1748–1846.* Vol. 14. New York: AMS Press, 1966.

Twitchell, Ralph Emerson. *The Spanish Archives of New Mexico.* Santa Fe: New Mexico State Record Center and Archives, 1914.

United States Senate. *Journal of the Executive Proceedings of the Senate of the United States of America, from the commencement of the First, to the termination of the Nineteenth Congress.* Vol. 3. Washington, D.C.: Duff Green, 1828.

———. "Answers of Augustus Storrs, of Missouri, to Certain Queries upon the Origin, Present State and Future Prospects of Trade and Intercourse, between Missouri and the Internal Provinces of Mexico, Propounded by the Hon. Mr. [Thomas Hart] Benton, Jan. 3, 1825." Senate Document No. 7, 18th Congress, 2nd session. Washington, D.C.: Government Printing Office, 1825.

Valerio-Jiménez, Omar S. *River of Hope: Forging Identity and Nation in the Rio Grande Borderlands.* Durham, N.C.: Duke University Press, 2013.

Vázquez, Dizan. *Fundación de la Diócesis de Chihuahua y su primer Obispo.* Chihuahua: N.p., 2008.

Weber, David J. *The Extranjeros: Selected Documents from the Mexican Side of the Santa Fe Trail, 1825–1828.* Santa Fe: Stagecoach Press, 1967.

———. *The Mexican Frontier, 1821–1846: The American Southwest under Mexico.* Albuquerque: University of New Mexico Press, 1982.

———. *On the Edge of Empire: The Taos Hacienda of Los Martinez.* Santa Fe: Museum of New Mexico Press, 1996.

———. *Northern Mexico on the Eve of the United States Invasion.* New York: Arno Press, 1976.

———. *The Taos Trappers: The Fur Trade in the Far Southwest, 1540–1846.* Norman: University of Oklahoma Press, 1970.

———. "William Workman: A Letter from Taos, 1826." *New Mexico Historical Review* 41 (April 1966): 155–61.

———. "Señor Escudero Goes to Washington: Diplomacy, Indians and the Santa Fe Trade." *Western Historical Quarterly* 43, no. 4 (Winter 2012): 417–35.

Williams, Walter. *A History of Northeast Missouri.* Vol. 1. Chicago: Lewis, 1913.

Wilson, James Grant, and John Fiske, eds. *Appleton's Cyclopaedia of American Biography.* Vol. 2. New York: D. Appleton & Co., 1887.

Index